I'm Ralph,
I'm Dad

'In *I'm Ralph, I'm Dad* Dr Mafi uses her father's biography and practical examples of his life with dementia, to show that identity, humour and spirituality are retained even late in the illness. Glennis reveals the beauty of every-day existence when caring for someone with this disability and the importance of 'being a friend of time' in this situation. Family photos and sketches enhance the gentle words. This book will greatly comfort people afraid of dementia, whether for themselves or others.'

– Dr Chris Perkins (FRNZCP, Psychiatrist of Old Age)

'Dementia is a deep, complex and meaningful experience. Its presence reminds us that we are much more than our memories. We are human beings who live in bodies that are weak and broken, but sometimes that brokenness can help us to see the world a little more clearly. To be human is to have a body, not just a brain. To be human is to be loved in community; to be loved by God and by one another. It is love that defines our humanness, not our abilities to remember things or to think clearly. Glennis Mafi offers an important insight into dementia in all of its dimensions – physical, spiritual and relational. She draws us towards that strange new world of dementia, not in a spirit of fear, but in a spirit of love, hope and new possibilities. If we can look differently at dementia then perhaps we can care more passionately. This book will help us move onto the road towards such a goal.'

– John Swinton (Professor of practical theology and pastoral care at the University of Aberdeen, Scotland)

I'm Ralph, I'm Dad

by **DR GLENNIS MAFI**

A Daughter Explores Identity,
Relationship and a Gentler Dementia

I'm Ralph, I'm Dad
Published by Glennis Mafi
with Rampart Publishing
(an imprint of Castle Publishing Ltd)
New Zealand

© 2020 Glennis Mafi
glennis.books@gmail.com

ISBN 978-0-473-51866-0 (Softcover)
ISBN 978-0-473-51867-7 (ePUB)
ISBN 978-0-473-51868-4 (Kindle)

Editing:
Andrea Candy

Illustration:
Graham Braddock

Production & Typesetting:
Andrew Killick
Castle Publishing Services
www.castlepublishing.co.nz

Cover design:
Paul Smith

About the cover: Dementia stole Ralph's capacity to engage fully
in family events, but surrounded by loving family (here his sister, a son,
two daughters and a granddaughter) and able to remain in
pleasant surroundings, a gently glowing joy and hope eased the journey.

Dedicated to my father, Ralph Wood,
who in his dementia taught us how to
live in the moment and remained Ralph and Dad
right up to that last wink!

Foreword

IN MY OPINION, this small book is destined to have an impact on the world of dementia that is considerably greater than its size might suggest possible. I use the term 'world of dementia' advisedly because it has implications for both the personal care of individuals with dementia and the way in which psychologists and other professionals think about people with dementia in general.

When I was a medical student in the 1950s, dementia was a relatively uncommon condition, usually referred to as 'senile dementia'. Lord Russell Brain's authoritative textbook, *Clinical Neurology*, of 1960 devoted just one page out of 400 to the dementias; one line to Alzheimer's disease. But with the ageing of populations – incidentally generally considered to be a 'good thing' – the incidence of dementia also rose. It became apparent that old age and dementia are concomitant phenomena.

This observation was scary enough to persuade the powers that be to provide greater resources for the study of phenomena in the brain that are responsible for the deterioration in memory, intellect and social functions that characterise dementias. Some of the world's most advanced research which is changing the way we think about the brain is being carried out in New Zealand. This book is not a textbook of medicine, but Dr Mafi does briefly refer to new evidence that is emerging. For example, as medical students we were taught that the tissues of the brain, once damaged, were unable to regenerate and that brain cells have specificity of function. But we now know that neither is correct. It has been found that brain tissues have a certain 'plasticity', meaning that they can take over the role of other, damaged cells. The research has not as yet produced a 'cure' or even yet a credible delaying of the onset of Alzheimer's disease, but important progress is being made. Not the least is the finding that Alzheimer's disease, although important numerically, is only one of some 40 causes of dementia. Some of these can, in fact, be treated.

It wasn't only doctors who felt the pressure of increasing numbers of aged people with dementia. Until the 1970s most of these people were cared for at home. Then as the levels of dementia increased, the complexity of their care needs also increased, but few caregivers have suitable training. In some cases, caregivers are obliged to leave paid employment because of the clash of responsibilities. Others find themselves precipitated into caring for their elderly relations while also retaining responsibility for their own children. This causes resentment, especially if the load falls on one family member. In research carried out in the 1980s by my unit at the University of Auckland, it was found that there were high levels of anger and depression among caregivers. Some openly confessed to sometimes wishing the recipient of their care was dead. To make matters worse, there was little access to respite care – or 'time off' for the caregivers. Meanwhile, the community regarded dementia as a social stigma, in much the way that it regarded schizophrenia, cerebral palsy and depression: an unfortunate condition to be kept out of sight.

Concern about the possibility of a major 'blow out' in the health budget, due to the need for care for increasing numbers of people with dementia, led to a move by several philosophers of a liberal bent to promote a new ethical approach to the distribution of resources. They began by developing a theory of 'personhood', which stated that only an individual who exhibits self-awareness or 'sentience' should be defined as a 'person'. And only a person should be guaranteed the protection of society, including life itself. Such a definition taken to its logical conclusion puts at risk new-born babies, people with a variety of cerebral palsies and congenital and acquired neurological conditions, anyone who becomes comatose and those with dementia. This philosophy also undergirds the legalisation of euthanasia and justifies the side-lining of people with dementia in poorly equipped nursing homes and dementia units. Many have been effectively abandoned by their families.

Although the passage of time has seen some relaxation in society's attitudes to dementia, there remains a vocal group that considers the most 'compassionate' way to manage people with dementia is by way of euthanasia, with or without a request. This despite the setting up of specialised geriatric and psychogeriatric services, the increasing sophistication of community nursing services and great improvements in residential care facilities.

Be that as it may, Dr Mafi, in the light of her own experience with a much-loved father with dementia, takes a major step up as she recounts how she retained coherent communication with him for as long as possible. She agrees with researchers such as John Swinton that much of a sufferer's persona is actually due to the labels applied by other people, rather than a function of the disease itself. She discovers the value of past memories of family life, humour, music and what her dad can still access of his own spiritual journey to create tranquillity. She finds that, even in what turned out to be her dad's last days, there are sparks of understanding and self-expression that remind her that he is more than a cipher – he is a being with personality and still capable of showing it.

This volume maintains its readers' interest from beginning to end. The combination of Dr Mafi's original poetry, her brother Graham Braddock's exceedingly apt illustrations and the explanatory material that holds the narrative together combine to make it not just a manual on dementia, but a great read in its own right.

Dr David E. Richmond
Professor Emeritus
Geriatric Medicine
University of Auckland

Contents

Preface

I NEVER PLANNED to write a book about dementia, or a book about my father Ralph Wood. But on one occasion, having spent an evening as his caregiver, I tried to step back, observe, and write a poem about our time together ('Dad-sitter'). Later I wrote more poems, finding, in a funny kind of way, that it lightened the load and the sorrow of watching my father slip further and further into full-blown dementia. My family enjoyed the poems, and I began to notice that many of them illustrated features of dementia and could be woven into a practical and informative commentary about the disease.

So my first thanks go to Dad himself who never knew he would become 'famous' in this way. However, he heard some of the poems and I think appreciated them. I still remember the funny face he pulled when I read 'Pooh Corner' to him. He and my mother Hazel always encouraged me in every endeavour in my life, and I am sure would have given their approval for a part of their story to be shared with others who find themselves caught up in the dementia experience.

Many people have cheered me on as I've worked on this book and in particular my sincere appreciation goes to:

Graham Braddock, my brother and well-known artist, for the

heart-warmingly, true-to-life illustrations which are based on photos of Dad.

My husband Manu and all my family members, for appreciating my poems and encouraging me.

My son David Mafi and his wife Marcelle, Dad's main caregivers for his last two and a half years, for taking photos of Dad at home and passing on his comical comments.

Ainslie Wood, Dad's sister, for filling in some gaps in his life story and supplying photos.

Sylvia Coulter, my English teacher sister, for encouragement and proofreading.

Sister-in-law Joan Braddock, already in print herself, for many valuable ideas and advice.

Emeritus Professor Dr David Richmond for his thoughtful and encouraging foreword.

Dr John Swinton, Professor of Practical Theology and Pastoral Care at the University of Aberdeen, Scotland, whom I met at a symposium on Disability and the Christian Church and whose book *Dementia: Living in the Memories of God*, opened up for me a vast new landscape of ideas related to dementia.

Dr Mary Tucker, one-time lecturer for the Postgraduate Diploma of Geriatrics at the University of Auckland, for advising on the medical content.

Dr Phil Wood, geriatrician and lead physician for the Memory Clinic at North Shore Hospital, Auckland, for advice in the care of Dad during his dementia and helpful suggestions when he reviewed my book.

Andrew Killick of Castle Publishing who, with great patience and knowledge, has guided me through this first-time experience of publishing a book.

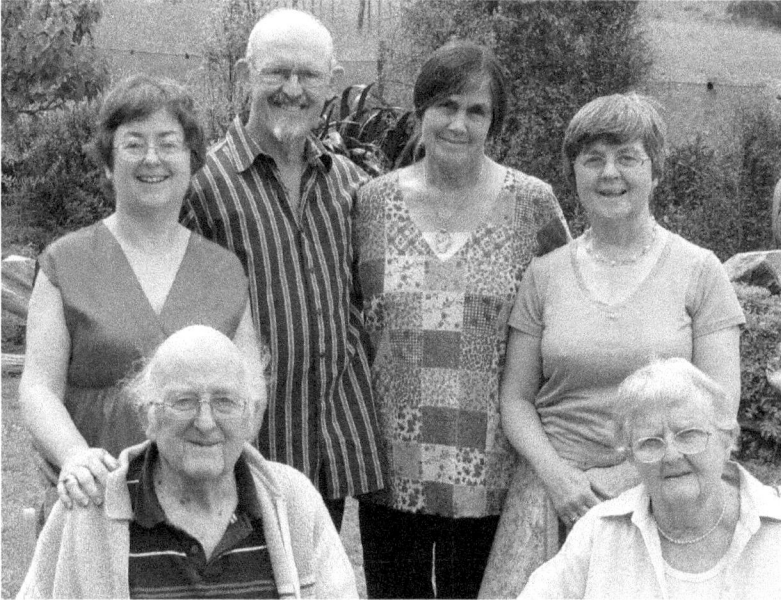

Ralph and family.
Back: Glennis (daughter), Graham (son), Joan (daughter-in-law)
and Sylvia (daughter). Front: Ralph and Ainslie (sister).

Disclaimer: I have taken care to ensure that the information about dementia is accurate at the time of writing, but knowledge about dementia is constantly changing as new research and observations come to light. Also, this is my father's story alone. Dementia will always be a little different in each affected person even though there may be common patterns. In addition, the poet in me just had to insert a little bit of imagination and speculation here and there as I tried to understand what was going on inside my father's mind. If you have specific questions about dementia in yourself or a loved one, please take them to an appropriate health professional.

Introduction

DEMENTIA. It's a huge topic which is examined, tossed around, talked about, feared and tackled by so many groups in society, from government ministries, medical specialists, economists and journalists to support groups, families and individuals. As a general practitioner (family doctor) I had patients with dementia, and I have read about and studied it, but the whole topic took quite a different turn for me when my own father, Ralph Wood, began to show the signs of dementia.

Dementia comes on slowly and insidiously. (For a formal definition of dementia see Appendix 1.) It doesn't have a clear or abrupt start like a stroke. Everyone is busily getting on with their lives, and slowly it dawns that Dad, Grandma or spouse keeps forgetting things, asks the same questions over and over, can't complete a simple task, gets lost in familiar territory, and so on. Everyone, including the family and the sufferer, tries to compensate or even cover up. A diagnosis is eventually made and outside help marshalled. And the disease progresses inexorably, as an example from my father illustrates. At first, we could leave Dad alone at home for a while with a prepared snack and everything he needed for a cup of tea laid out beside the electric jug, and he would look after himself. Later, he had trouble working out how to make the cup of tea; then he wouldn't think to stand up and get the snack and eat it. He'd just sit. Later again, he would even need prompting to drink the cup of tea in front of him.

≈

Cup of Tea for Dad

Tea, big cup, strong with milk and sugar,
as he relaxes down on the garden seat,
removes his cap and scratches his sweaty pate.

Tea, no milk, and no sugar,
for heart health, they say.
'I don't know, Ralph, these cups do stain so!'

Waking-up-tea, in fine china 'Father' cup
as he sits in bed with Hazel,
plaid capes draped around their scrawny shoulders.

'Tea's by the kettle Dad, just add boiling water,
and there's bikkies on the plate...'
while we rush off, wondering if he'll remember.

Tea going cold, forgotten...
'Drink it up, Dad.'
And he sits, immobile, staring into the blank page
of another today.

'Tea tempers the spirit and harmonises the mind, dispels

lassitude and relieves fatigue, awakens thought and prevents drowsiness, lightens or refreshes the body, and clears the perceptive faculties.[1] Wish it was true, Dad!

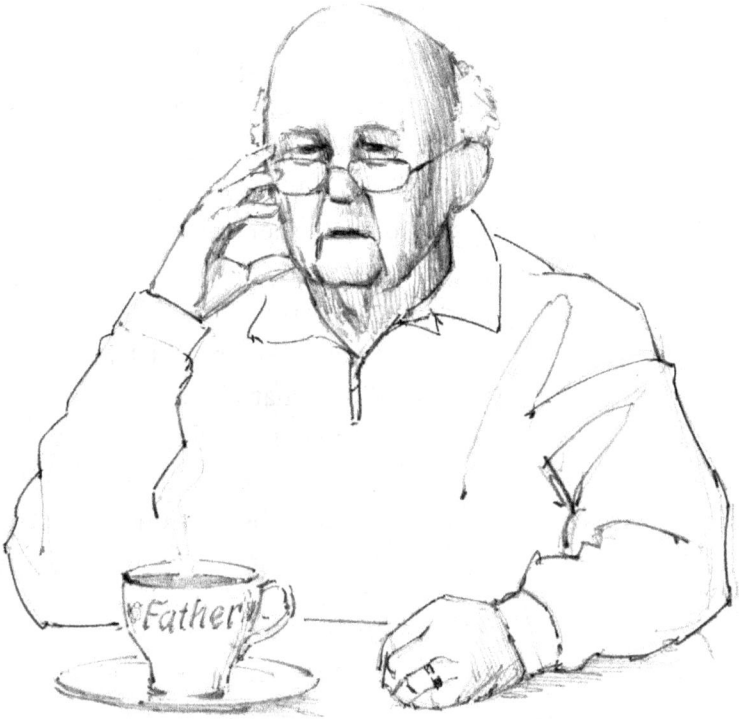

Increasingly, Dad retreated into a world of his own where ordinary communication and stimuli hardly seemed to register with him, and conversely, very little communication or activity was initiated by him. But every now and then he surprised us

1. Confucius, quoted on a Dilmah cup.

with a wry comment, an animated facial expression, or unexpectedly energetic action. On one occasion, some young people were singing a lively song, and as I walked out of the room with Dad he did a brief little tap dance with his feet and his stick. Sometimes it was a smile and an inappropriately loud 'Hello' in church when great-grandchild Judah walked up beside him. Then there was the visit to the audiologist. As she began to inspect Dad's ears with the auriscope, he asked her what she was doing. She told him she was checking his ears and jokingly said she wanted to know if she could see through to the other side! He put his hand up beside the other ear, waved it and with a funny smile said, 'I'm waving at you!'

As I noticed these things, observing the fluctuating but slowly progressive course of Dad's dementia, I tried to look beyond his daily needs to work out what was really going on in his mind and to express this in poems. As I have reflected on these last years of his life, it appears to me that 'Dementia Dealt Gently' with him and the poems and observations hint at why this was so.

A Short Biography of
Ralph Alveston Wood

M Y FATHER, RALPH WOOD, was born in 1924 and grew up in Devonport on Auckland's North Shore, with father Harold, mother Nellie, big brother Alan, young brother Neil, and little sister Ainslie. Their concrete house was the last on the left in Ngataringa Road. It had a big garden and backed onto the bay. It was aptly named 'The Moorings' because at the bottom of the zig-zag path down the cliff was a tiny beach, a boat slip and a boat shed where the family yacht and dinghy were kept. Other members of the large Wood family lived in Devonport and many of them were also into yachting, so it is no wonder that sailing seemed to be in Ralph's blood. He learnt yachting skills at a young age when they sailed down the harbour or up to the family bach at Paremoremo. Dad's father was a plumber and is said to have cycled to a job balancing a gas stove on his bicycle, a skill apparently picked up by his son Ralph who I've been told biked (or more realistically walked) home from Takapuna Grammar with the desk he had made at woodwork also balanced on his bike!

Harold died when Ralph was just fourteen, and Nellie must have struggled at times to bring up her four children. But they all helped, and perhaps that is one of the reasons Dad was so practical, developing home handyman skills and a love of

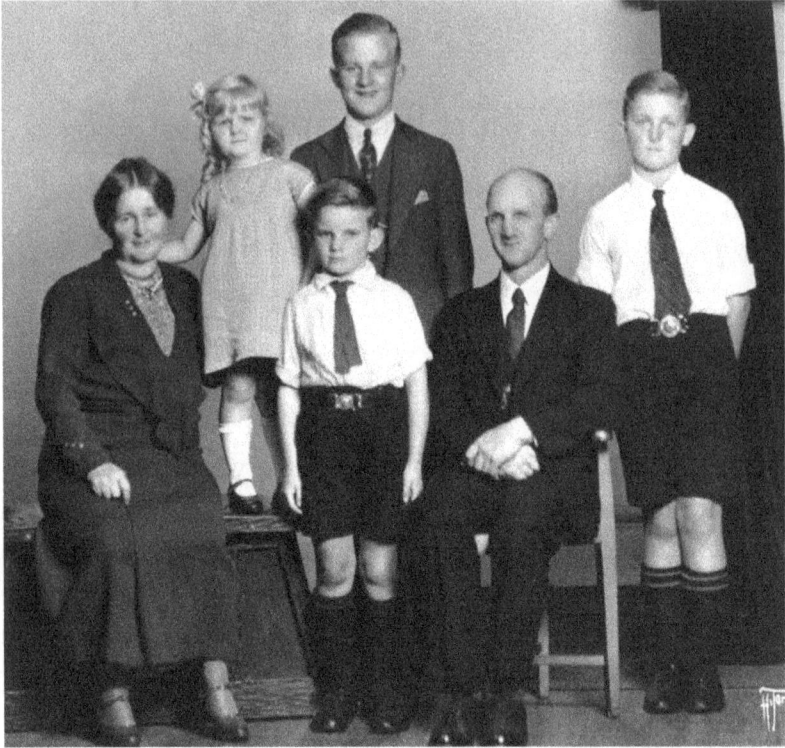

Ralph's family. Nellie, Ainslie, Neil (in front), Alan (behind), Harold and Ralph.

gardening. The Moorings garden was large, with fruit trees, grapevines, vegetables, tangled Cape gooseberry bushes and an A-framed moveable chicken coop. Even in my time, I remember Grandma's homemade bars of soap and tins of baked bread 'biscuits', evidence of the thrifty ways she used to survive with her family.

After four years at Takapuna Grammar, Dad studied accounting at night school while working at the Guardian Trust. In November 1945 Ralph, aged twenty-one, married Hazel Braddock

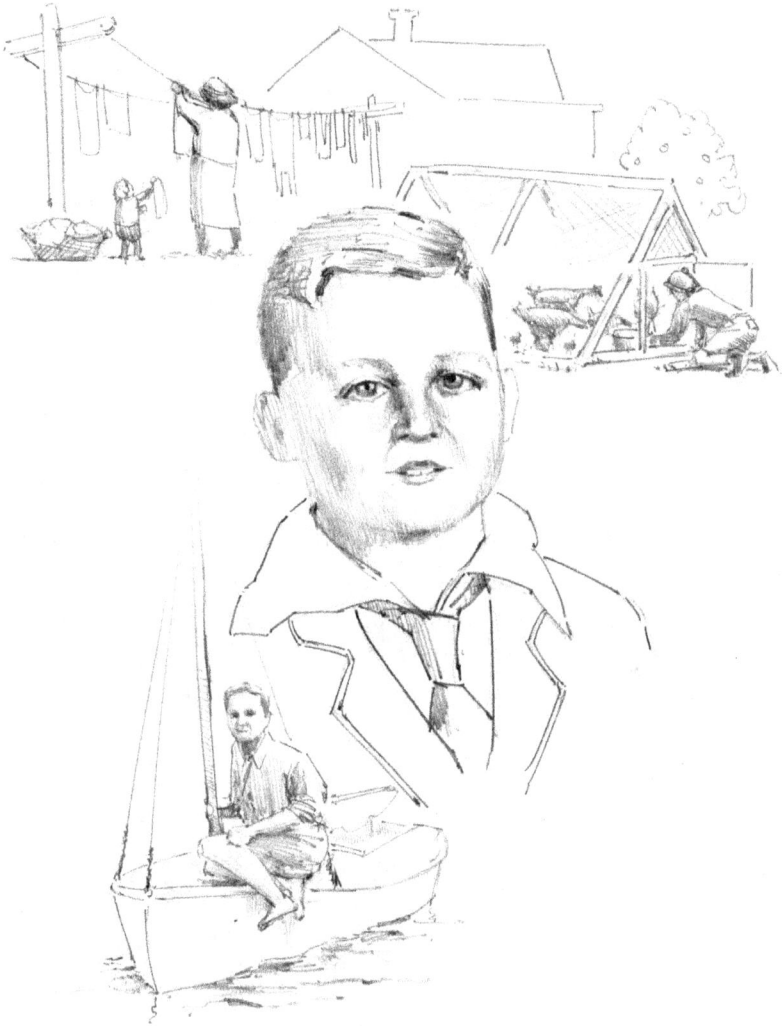

(née Penman) a twenty-six-year-old widow with a three-year-old son. Both had already suffered tragic losses in their lives. Ralph had seen his dad struggle for breath as he died of pneumonia. A few years later Neil developed a mental illness which at that time carried a heavy stigma. With Neil incarcerated in a mental asylum, and subdued with the unpleasant medications of the time, Ralph apparently tucked him away in a cloistered back recess of his mind, not to be included in real life. As for Hazel – her only sibling, a baby sister, died at eighteen months from pneumonia, a dreaded scourge in those pre-antibiotic days. Hazel was nine years old and still spoke of this sadness in her old age. In 1938, Hazel had married Maurice Braddock, but in 1942 as a conscientious objector under great pressure from the authorities and many others in society, he had committed suicide. Baby Graham was six months old. Hazel's grief must have been dreadful, although I hardly remember her talking about it. Perhaps it was just too hard. Instead, my overriding impression of my mother was the enthusiastic, fully involved joy she brought into her life and all her relationships.

The new marriage brought happiness, with Ralph becoming a steady and loving father for Graham. They had three more children, Sylvia, Glennis and David, while establishing their home in Harbour View Road, Pt Chevalier, a property which backed onto the tidal upper Waitemata Harbour, much like the old home at Devonport. They enjoyed gardening and keeping hens, tennis, swimming, making home movies, camping holidays and the family bach in the Waitakeres, while Dad was developing his own accountancy business. Many years were to go by before Dad could afford a yacht again, and then he opted for the convenience and versatility of a trailer-sailer.[2] Christian faith was a dominant part of Dad's life. Over the years he played many roles in church life, and in the family he led by example,

---

2. A yacht with retractable centreboard instead of a fixed keel, so it can be hauled out of the water and transported on a yacht trailer.

coaching us in Bible reading, memorising verses and regular church attendance.

Although Hazel was five years Ralph's senior, her sunny nature, active habits and youthful figure meant most people didn't know it, especially after Ralph went bald prematurely. However, their personalities were quite different and this could sometimes cause tension. Hazel, a much-loved only child, was confident and somewhat bossy. Dad had a quieter personality. When his father died, his mother had naturally tended to look to Alan to take the lead in some of the male roles in the family, and Ralph took on a more submissive support role. This carried into the marriage, where Mum seemed to make many of the day-to-day decisions and could get impatient if Dad was slow to speak up on an idea that needed a response. She did much of the organising of the family and household though Dad was perfectly capable in his accountancy business and his special interests like the garden and yachting. I refer to this in the poem, 'When did it Start?' because in his dementia, he quickly became very dependent on others to tell him what to do. This was partly due to his type of dementia, but his life experiences and personality no doubt also played a role.

Nevertheless, Mum was a cheerful and faithful encourager of Dad in many of his roles. She obviously loved him and wanted to build him up. Dad used to arrive home from work by bus at about the same time every evening, and a few minutes before he was expected, Mum would take off her apron, rush to the bathroom to tidy her hair and dab on a little rouge and lipstick before hurrying to the door to welcome him with her typical enthusiastic smile and matching body language.

They faced more sorrow when our happy family life was shattered by the untimely death of David in a road accident, two days before his fourteenth birthday. Later, their attentive son-in-law Aubrey died too young of a brain tumour, and just eleven months after that, Aubrey and Sylvia's son Hamish died in an avalanche on Mt Ruapehu. Dad seemed to absorb these tragedies into himself and didn't say much or express his grief obviously as Mum did. She became depressed for some months after David's death, but her personality and her Christian faith wouldn't let her stay down for long. Somehow, together, Mum and Dad were able to weather life's sorrows.

Ralph and Hazel were married for nearly sixty-one years. They didn't always agree, tempers flared sometimes, and they didn't share all the same interests or tastes, but their commitment to each other was unwavering. Overall, it was a good marriage. While their personalities and approach to life contrasted, they complemented each other well. Dad's retirement was gradual, and around that time they had the challenge and enjoyment of building and setting up a new house and property at Greenhithe on Auckland's North Shore. They enjoyed warm companionship as they developed their garden and shared family times with grandchildren and the growing tribe of great-grandchildren. They went for holidays in the yacht and later in their little campervan, and they visited me and my family in Tonga, often helping with the maintenance and decorating of our big house and medical clinic.

Dementia presents in different ways. With Dad's vascular (or possibly mixed) dementia there was less of the agitation, restlessness and aggression that is common in Alzheimer's dementia, and more passivity. He became increasingly inactive and passive, so that he needed to be prompted to do even quite simple tasks like putting on each article of clothing, eating his dinner, keeping on walking in a certain direction, and so on.

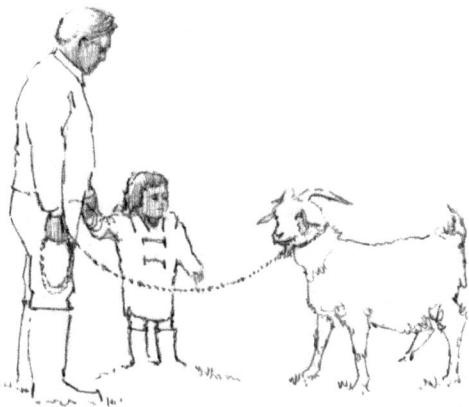

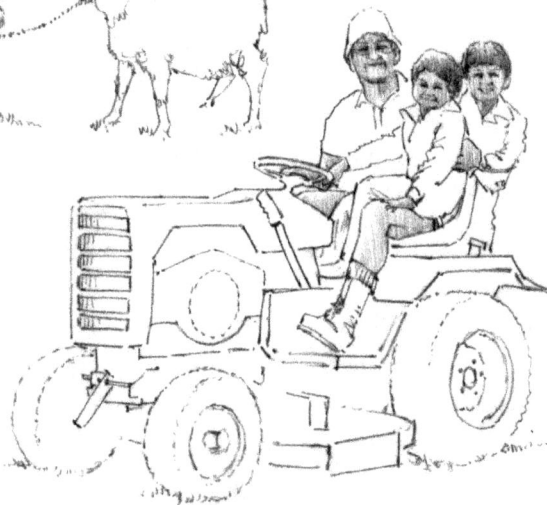

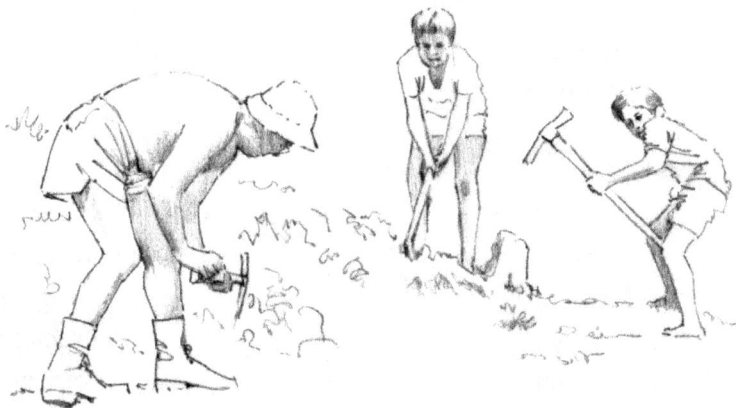

But life's experiences must also have a huge influence on the expression of dementia, and it is very possible that the quality of relationships with significant others such as a spouse or close partner play a part too. When he was well into his dementia we came to realise that although he could hardly explain what he was feeling, he was almost certainly depressed and that this was probably related to the loss of Hazel. She had walked alongside Ralph through sixty and a half years and no doubt was part of the reason 'Dementia Dealt Gently'.

During the last two to three years when his dementia was advanced, Dad had the privilege of remaining in his own home, cared for mainly by family members. Granddaughter Geraldine and her husband Jarrod lived in for four months, then grandson David and his wife Marcelle stayed for the last two and a half years. Funded caregivers, family members and friends all took their turn at Dad-sitting. He regularly spent a few hours two days a week at a local rest home, where he also slept over from time to time when we all had pressing engagements. This was a wonderful arrangement, allowing him to enjoy the familiar surroundings of home with loving family members, including two little great-grandchildren, while having regular respite care.

Dad's final illness lasted about three weeks, and during that time it was his memory of his wife, and of the Scriptures – so precious to him – which remained. On one occasion as he held my hand, he looked into my eyes and said, 'My dear wife Hazel.' I didn't mind the mistaken identity! On another occasion, when I said it was time for me to leave and was there anything he wanted, he simply said, 'The Lord is my Shepherd.' So I recited that beautiful psalm to him, especially noting the poignant assertion, 'Even though I walk through the valley of the shadow of death, I will fear no evil; for you are with me; your rod and your staff, they comfort me.'[3] Dad passed away peacefully a few days later on 1 June 2009 with four members of the family by his side.

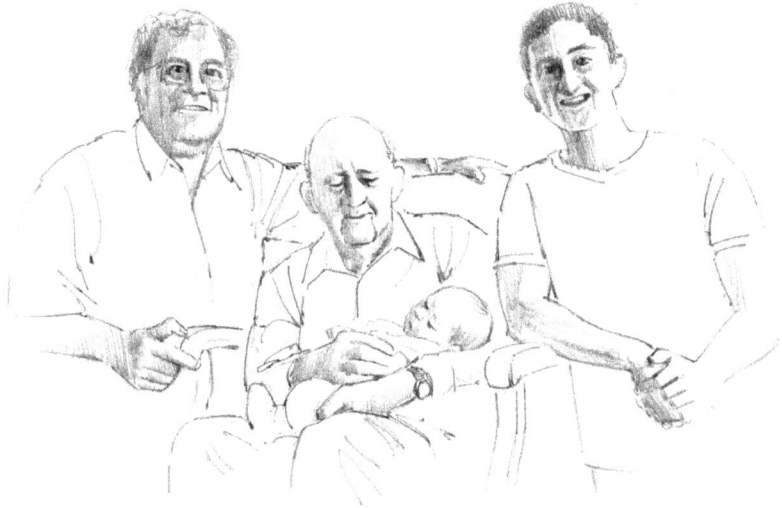

---

3. Psalm 23:4, *The Bible*.

Identity

Dad-sitting

I was Dad-sitting tonight.

We had a quiet evening.

He dawdled through his dinner
    while I finished mine and tidied the kitchen.
I tried to engage him in conversation,
    but we never got beyond a sentence or two.
I told him about the V8 car racing in Hamilton,
    and his still-accountant's mind asked how much they paid!
I trimmed his hair – so fine, like a baby's –
    (it was Mum's last instruction, 'Remember to cut Dad's hair.')
We listened to Saturday Night Requests – old-fashioned songs,
rag-time.
I danced crazily to one of them and he even tapped his feet
    (when I suggested it).
I played 'Moonlight Sonata' on the table-top and told him it was
easier than on the piano.
    He told me I was cheating.

I'm Ralph, I'm Dad

I gave him his pills, guided him through – teeth-cleaning,
                  – toilet
             – pyjamas
           – goodnight prayer and a kiss.

Yes, we had a quiet evening,
A no-work-done evening.

A wasted evening?

A memorable evening!

That moment of the special little gesture;
that spark of a mind not yet quite detached
when he put his arm around me – and patted my back.

Yes, that moment,

when the Dad-sat became the Daughter-sitter.

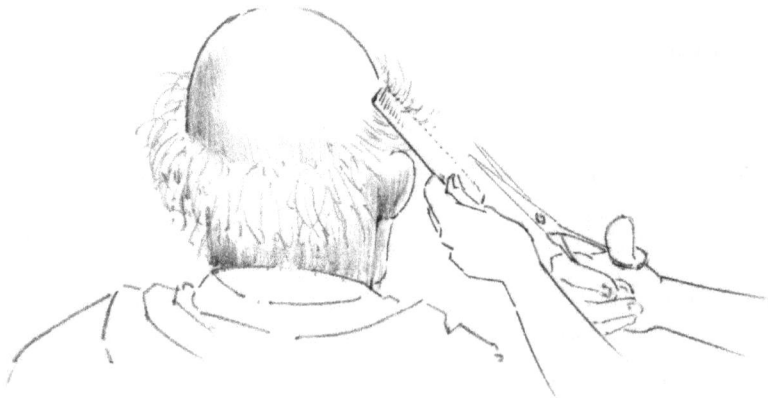

D EMENTIA COMES ON SLOWLY and in different ways in different people, so it can be difficult to diagnose. People with dementia also require a lot of care, though it varies greatly from person to person and over time as the disease progresses. (See Appendix 2 regarding early signs of dementia and the importance of ruling out other medical conditions.)

Ralph became increasingly inactive and passive, and could easily be 'forgotten'. He could be left having a rest on his bed while his caregivers pressed on with the many demands of their busy lives. Dad-sitter was my first poem about Dad, and it brought home to me not only that he still knew and loved me as his daughter but also the importance of spending time with Dad and not seeing it as 'wasted time', or feeling frustrated about all the other activities I had to forgo. For the few years he would be in this phase of his life, I needed to somehow rearrange my life to fit him in. Having several caregivers and extra friends and supporters who could take a turn with Dad made the process easier. I began to discover that with the right attitude, time can 'expand' and accommodate all that is truly needed.

John Swinton, in his book *Dementia: Living in the Memories of God*, brings out the idea of being friends of time, pointing out that 'many of us spend much of our lives at war with time.'[4] He includes two insightful quotes: 'The friend of time doesn't spend all day saying: 'I haven't got time.' He doesn't fight with time. He accepts it and cherishes it.'[5] And, 'To become a friend

---

4. John Swinton, *Dementia: Living in the Memories of God*, Grand Rapids, MI: W. B. Eerdmans, 2012, p.229.

5. Ibid, p.227. Quote from Jean Vanier, founder of L'Arche, an International Federation of communities for people with intellectual and developmental disabilities, and those who assist them.

of someone with Alzheimer's, I think, is exactly the kind of challenge that it means to become a friend of time. We forget that our most precious gift for others is presence; just being present... When there is not a lot to do other than to be present, you find out... what it means to be a friend of time.'[6]

---

6. Swinton, *Dementia: Living in the Memories of God*, p.229. Quote from Stanley Hauerwas, *There is a Bridge*, DVD.

When Did It Start?

When did it start – this dementia?
　　This dream existence descending on him,
　　these doldrums settling over Dad's mind,
　　the sails limp, the boat going nowhere?

Did it start years ago when he was slow to answer?
　　When Mum made the daily decisions?
　　Or was that his after work wind-down,
　　knowing she had it under control?

Did it start when he passively accepted
　　her busy meeting of his needs?
　　Or after all those years had she become
　　the wind beneath his sails?

Was it starting when he couldn't remember
　　who was who in Coronation Street,
　　and Mum grew impatient with
　　explaining over and over?

Surely it was starting
　　when he had the stroke,[7]
　　and the CT scan showed
　　'mild frontal lobe atrophy'?

7.　In 1997, when he was aged 73.

And it was well underway when he
    kept asking the same question,
    and Mum had to restrain her tongue
    and grow her patience.

Yes, it had him for sure when Mum
    fell and broke her hip,
    and he couldn't understand to find the alarm[8]
    and press the button.

He didn't have a family history.
    He never smoked,
        took no alcohol.
            He was intelligent,
                used his brain actively.
                He was sociable,
                    had overall good health.

So why? How? ...Will it happen to me?

Don't fret about it.
    Take off the label, the D word, Dementia.
    It's not so bad!

So Dad's brain is wearing out before his joints,
    his memory before his heart.
    So what?
    He's still Dad – and we love him!

---

8. A medical alarm for summoning help.

WHY DID MY FATHER get dementia? When did it start? Should I have had him checked out sooner? Is it starting in my brain? Such questions are understandably asked by family, friends and early sufferers of dementia.

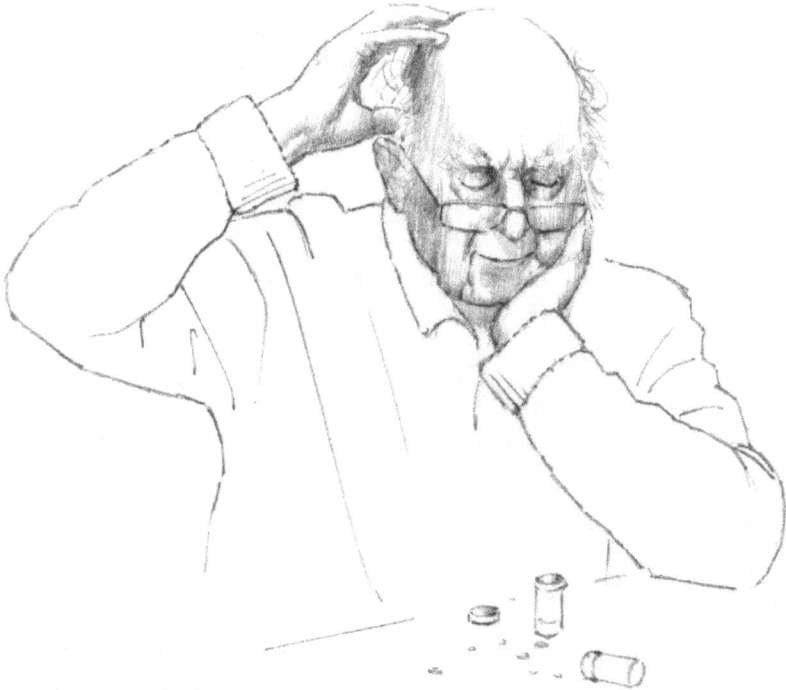

Overall, we don't really know why this person gets dementia and not that one, and a genetic link is not fully proven except in a few rarer types of dementia. Its gradual onset makes a start date impossible to apply. Despite that, an early diagnosis, though distressing, can be very useful, enabling the person and the person's family to complete legal matters such as a will, advanced care planning, and enduring power of attorney. A savvy person with a new diagnosis of dementia may be able to do much sat-isfying preparation, simplifying, adapting, socialising and even making active contributions to the world of dementia research, education and support. An inspiring example of this is told by Wendy Mitchell in her book *Somebody I Used to Know*, written after she was given a diagnosis of early onset dementia.[9]

There is more detail in Appendix 3 about risk factors for dementia and how we can help ourselves prevent or delay it.

The definition of dementia and its various types is useful for doctors, lawyers and researchers, but it describes 'typical' pat-terns in 'typical' people. In real life, whatever is going on in the brain, Dad is still Dad, a unique person with his own personal experiences, feelings, loves and joys – it helps to hang on to this.[10] It is interesting that in the Tongan language there is no real word for dementia. When some of the signs of what we would label dementia began to be seen in some of my many older Tongan patients, the family carer would gently laugh and say, 'She's just forgetful, just getting old!' ('loto ngalongalo' in Tongan, meaning 'forgetful') and carry on loving, respecting and assisting her as they would for any older family member without thinking there was a disease to be considered.

This poem also raises the sense of fear which is very common with regard to dementia.[11] We fear that in losing our memory

---

9. Wendy Mitchell with Anne Wharton, *Somebody I Used to Know*, London, UK: Bloomsbury, 2018.

10. Swinton has an interesting discussion around the purpose and limitation of definitions in psychiatric and neurological conditions such as dementia in *Dementia: Living in the Memories of God*, 2012, p.33-46.

11. In a British YouGov poll of 2000 people in the United Kingdom,

and our capacity to think and reason we will lose ourselves or become non-people. But it is not so. See Appendix 4 for a more reassuring look at what it really means to be human.

---

31 percent of respondents feared dementia the most, with 27 percent fearing cancer and 18 percent fearing death the most. Among retirees, 34 percent worry about health the most, specifically dementia (52 percent), cancer (33 percent) and stroke (3 percent). Alzheimer's Research UK quoted by Swinton, *Dementia: Living in the Memories of God*, 2012, p.187.

I'm Ralph, I'm Dad

Who am I?

They call me Ralph, and Dad.
There's something familiar about that
So I guess that's who I am.
　　But what am I doing?

Mostly I do what I'm told –
　　Stand up
　　Come through here
　　Sit down
　　Eat up!

They give the commands;
I try to process them
But my body is slow to respond.
　　Move to the right, they say,
　　Look, it's there on your right,
But my right isn't quite right![12]

So I'm eating marmalade toast.
Now that's familiar,
But what was I doing five minutes ago?

No continuity
Disjointed episodes of Now
No clear memories of Past
No memory of planned Future

---

12. Dad's stroke caused a right-sided hemianopia, meaning he couldn't see well on the right side.

Just Now
A Now I mostly can't understand
A Now I can rarely control.

Kind people come and go, some vaguely familiar,
All mixed up in the slowly swirling tangle of my mind,
Like an impossible jigsaw puzzle where pieces won't relate
Except here and there, at last, a match,
Like the photo of that handsome young lad –
I *knew* he was my son.[13]

I'm Ralph, I'm Dad – that's who I am.

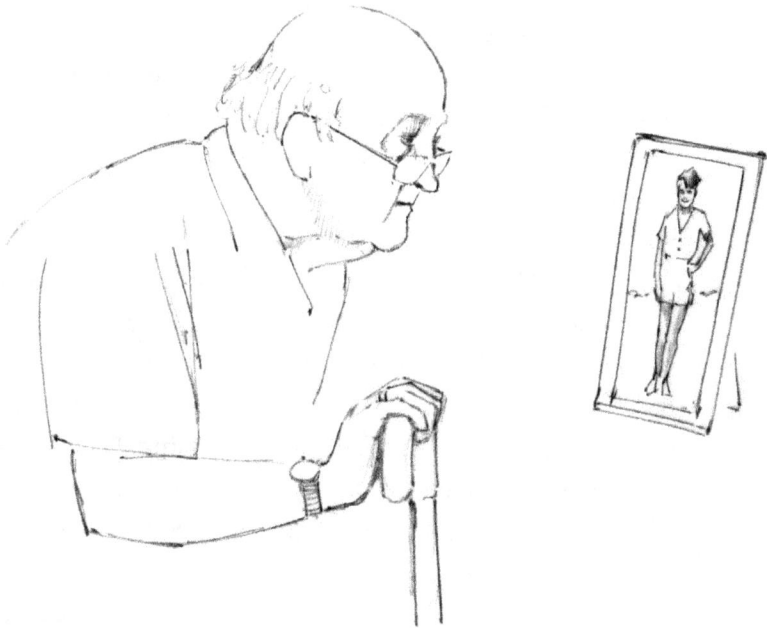

_____

13. Dad's son David had died forty-two years before, at the age of fourteen.

THIS POEM WAS AN ATTEMPT to try to get inside the mind of someone with dementia. Is it a confusing blur of thoughts and impressions? Is it dominated by sad, or angry, or frustrated feelings? Is it just a blank for hours on end? As I observed my father, it appeared to me that he was always in the Now, the Present, confined to a tiny prison of time rather like the spatial equivalent of a prison cell. There is no outlook; he sees neither forward nor backward, just the enclosing stone walls of his time prison. (However, it is interesting to read the accounts of younger people at the beginning of their early onset dementia who describe how their mind functions, what they have difficulty with, how they compensate, and how it fluctuates from day to day.)[14]

It is fascinating, horrible and sad, but I suspect it was not as horrible for Dad as it was for me. He seemed to have the capacity to enjoy the Present, if it was a pleasant Present, and he appeared to lack the insight to be greatly bothered by his short-term memory loss, at least at that stage of his dementia. If we referred to something pleasant that had happened an hour or two ago, like a visit from his sister Ainslie, we might say, 'Well, that was lovely of Ainslie to come and spend the morning with you.' Then he was likely to respond, 'I suppose it was, though I don't remember', and he could say that with a smile and not appear to be the least bothered by it. When his great-grandson came up to him with a toy, chattering and smiling, Dad would respond with a smile and enjoy playing with him for a while. He lived in the present with none of the worries about time which so often consume us in our busy lives.

Long-term memory fades more slowly than short-term

---

14. Mitchell, *Somebody I Used to Know*, many places through the text.

memory, and some of the most heart-warming times for family caregivers are when the person with dementia remembers something from long ago that you thought had been forgotten – like the example in 'Who Am I?'. Sadly, these moments gradually become less frequent, but looking at photos of people and places that have been important seems to bring joy. It may confirm the individual's personal identity as a valued human being, not in the usual way as a person with full mental faculty, but as someone in a human relationship, like father and son. It is also strangely satisfying for the friend who takes the time to sit and remember.

Swinton points out that, 'Memory is ... both internal and external. Some of it is held by the individual; some of it is held by her community; all of it is held by God. ...even in normal times some of our memories are outside of ourselves and often stored and told by others around us. And when some things about ourselves are far from clear in our own minds, we can experience a sense of self through the memories of us held by those around us, through the stories they tell about us. Memory, like mind and personhood, is corporate through and through.'[15]

An interesting idea about photos and memories that can be used by caregivers to create a 'present of the past' can be found in Appendix 5. And in Appendix 6, there is an example from Wendy Mitchell of how she safeguarded her photos for future use.

---

15. Swinton, *Dementia: Living in the Memories of God*, quote from p.221.

Surprise!

I'm eating my dinner, taking my time.
The folk around me are eating too,
  only they seem to talk more than they eat!
First one, then another.
The words fly back and forth at great speed,
  a cacophony of sound swirling around me.
Sometimes I think I catch a real word,
  and sometimes I speak up, contributing my take on it.
Then one of them will correct me and explain,
  but I see the others chuckling.
They're not unkind – I just missed the point – again.
I shrug my shoulders and raise my eyebrows.
What's the use?
Back to my dinner.

Glennis tries to include me in the conversation.
'It's a noisy table we have tonight, Dad,' she says.
'It's not the table,' I reply dryly.

There's a pause, then a surprised laugh.
They didn't think I could come out with something quite so apt!

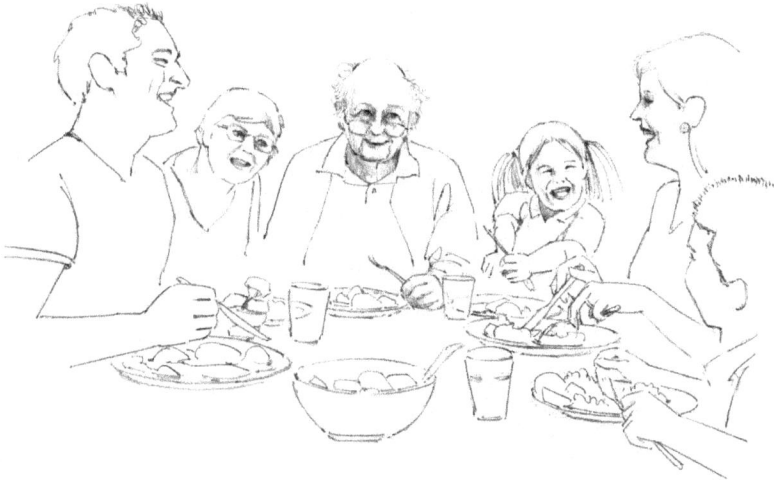

DAD'S DRY SENSE OF HUMOUR and tendency to come out with little puns and wisecracks stayed with him well into his dementia and helped us to remember he was still Dad with his own unique personality. Some of his plays on words were old favourites that he'd used many times before, like: 'I've got a backache [back cake] with no icing on it,' or when eating a fruit with seeds like a fig: 'Well, you're sure to succeed [suck seed].' When being told to put his hearing aid in, he might say, ''Ere, 'ere!' Or given his walking stick, he would tap it in a lively way and say, 'Ye old walking stick', or 'Jack Walker' referring to a long-deceased family connection. On one occasion, while a photo was being taken, the walking stick was used as a pretend gun, resulting in much hilarity.

Sometimes his witty responses took us by surprise, like the example in the poem. Another time, when I commented that his pills were running out, he replied, 'I didn't know I had athletic pills!' On another occasion, Dad and I were dining alone and in semi-formal style I said to him, 'Let us partake of our lettuce soup,' to which he replied, 'Then let us not delay the partakation.' And when I was encouraging him to join me in a hymn and read out the first line of the second verse: 'Great things he hath taught us...', he responded facetiously, 'Where's the tortoise?'

Personality does change with dementia. Previously warm and friendly people may become suspicious and even para-noid, but habitual thought patterns and personality traits will stay a long time – a sobering observation! Equally sobering is understanding that in dementia judgement, emotional con-trol and social behaviour may also deteriorate, especially in what is called frontotemporal dementia. With social control gone or inhibited, behaviours or thoughts normally hidden may come out, rather like someone under the influence of alcohol. Neuropsychologist Edward Welch writes of dementia, 'Whatever the person thought or did in private is now public, because the person does not distinguish between the two any longer... when we are intellectually less competent, some of these private events begin to slip out.'[16]

---

16. Edward T. Welch, *Blame it on the Brain?* Phillipsburg, N. J.: P & R Publishing, 1998, p.79 and pp.56-58. This is an older book first published in 1953 and written from a Christian counsellor's observa-tions. It would be interesting to research the content of what people with dementia say or do in relation to their characteristic thought patterns and behaviours for years before, including those politely hidden from public view. A lot of research has looked at the influ-ence of diet, lifestyle, education, etc. on the occurrence of dementia; so far I have not found research on what really influences content and behaviour in dementia, though there are some characteristic patterns in different types of dementia.

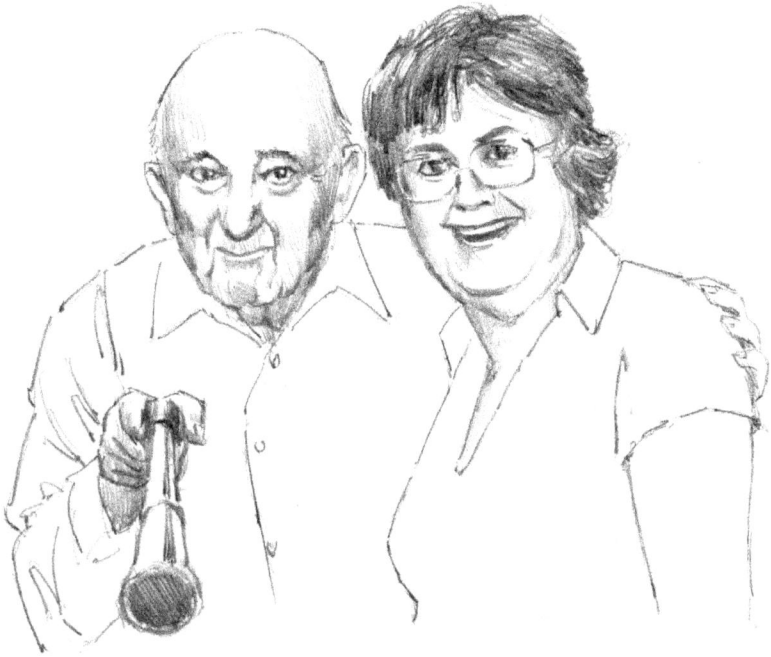

Father the Accountant

Father was a family man
    He loved his wife
    He loved his kids
    He cleaned up when we were sick
    He quizzed us for exams
    And he took us camping
        But mostly he was an accountant.

Father was a gardener
    He composted and mulched
    Tied tomatoes with flax string
    He grew beans, beets and carrots
    Braided onions in long ropes
    Stored kumara in sawdust
        But mostly he was an accountant.

Father was a handyman
    He plumbed and hammered
    He painted and wallpapered
    He made cupboards and fixed locks
    He built a bush cottage
    With a toilet that flushed
        But mostly he was an accountant.

Father was a seaside man
   He loved to swim and dive
   He swam with kids on his back
   He surfaced like a whale
   He towed us in a blown-up tyre
   And he sailed trailer-sailers
      But mostly he was an accountant.

First, he was a company accountant
And worked for other bosses.
Then he was a chartered accountant
And worked for himself – and for businesses
         societies
         churches
         friends
         family...

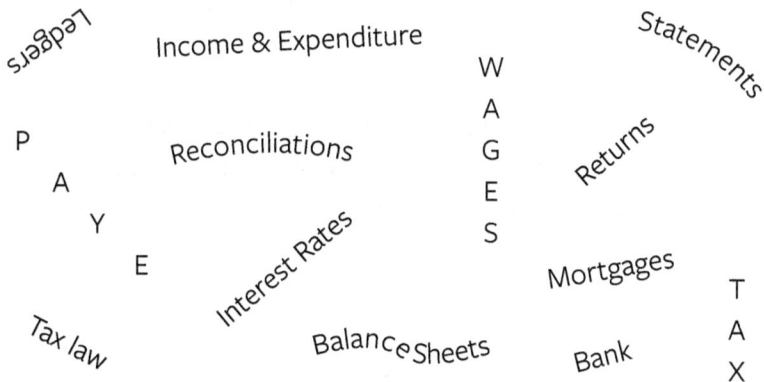

Ledgers   Income & Expenditure   Statements

P   Reconciliations   W A G E S   Returns

A

Y

E   Interest Rates   Mortgages

Tax law   Balance Sheets   Bank   T A X

I'm Ralph, I'm Dad

Now Father is an old man
    He's deaf and can't see well
    His memory's mostly gone
    He walks with shuffly gait
    He itches and he aches
    And numbers make him spin
        But he's still an accountant!

I've been to work today, Dad.
        How do they calculate your pay?

We'll have to buy you some new shoes, Dad.
        What about the budget?

Don't worry, Sylvia looks after your finances now.
        Has she completed the tax return?

Here's your dinner Dad.
        Have you paid the mortgage on the soup?

Will you say grace, Dad?
        Loving Heavenly Father, we are ever grateful for all your goodness and especially for the provision of this food. Bless it to our use, and may you bless this business so that we will sell everything that has to be sold!

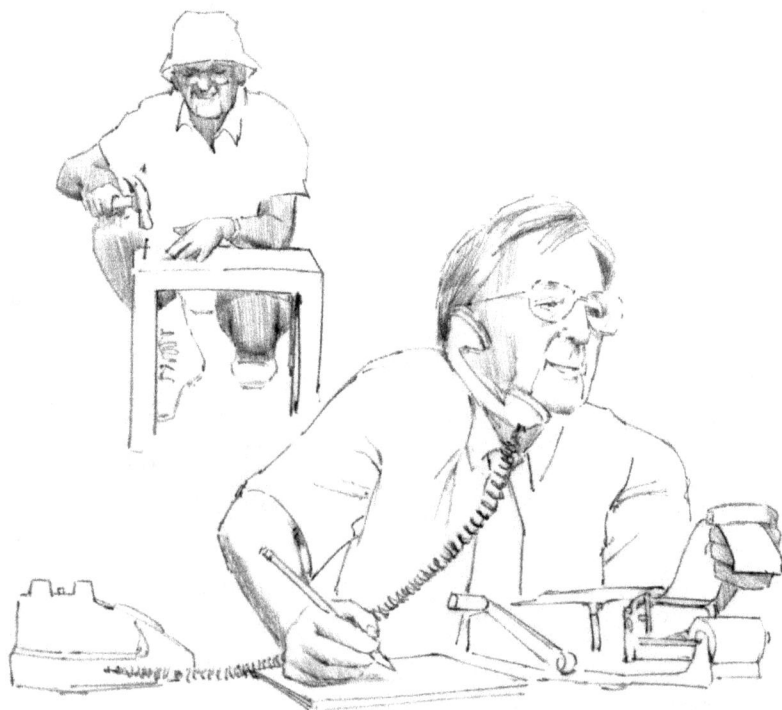

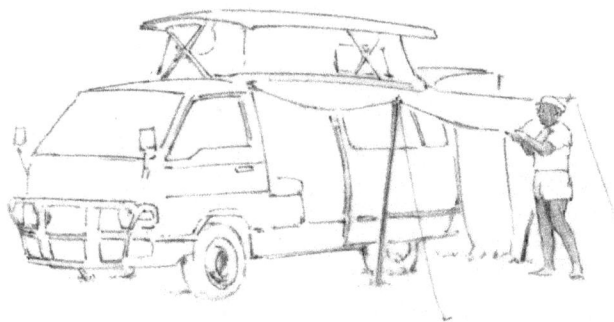

JUST AS PERSONALITY TRAITS can be recognised well into the dementia experience, so can the habits and training of years, and this can be used by insightful caregivers to assist with the care of their relative or client. In the rich tapestry of his life, Dad had many interests and skills, but his profession as an accountant obviously was deeply entrenched in his mind and memory so that accounting topics frequently entered into his talk and even his prayers. Talking about business, money, the financial situation and so on would also, at least for a while, provide him with the opportunity to be involved in a conversation that made some sense to him.

Finding out the employment history and previous interests of a person with dementia can foster understanding in the caregiver and even help with care. For example, one rest home attached a toy toolset to the bedroom door of a retired mechanic who tended to get lost, so he could recognise his room. Penny Garner calls this finding the 'Primary Theme', a 'narrative from the client's past that...will provide them with a continuing sense of achievement gained from a particular area of past expertise no matter how modest.'[17]

---

17. Oliver James, *Contented Dementia*, London: Vermilion, 2008, p.63 and elsewhere.

Swing-bed Yacht

Captain Ralph is at the tiller,
Swing-bed Yacht rocks in the bay,
Crewman Judah laughs and squeals
Then – splash! – he swims away!

Ralph's first yacht was the Daisy
(I'm sure I've heard him say),
She set his sail on yachting
In Ngataringa Bay.

See, sailing was a family thing
Upstream to Lucas Creek,
Or down the gulf in uncle's yacht
The fresh sea-breeze to seek.

Then after years of labour
Four kids, lush garden, chooks,
Dream took shape in trailer-sailer
Wooed him from accounting books.

The 'Rosalind', his pride and joy,
Her sails flap, then fill,
We skim along by nature's power,
Exhilaration, thrill!

And even Mum set fears aside
And joined him as first hand
Their many holidays were blessed –
Fresh wind and waves and sand.

I'm Ralph, I'm Dad

But Time, relentless, stalked him down
The fate of all mankind.
Heart failed, mind slowed, stroke struck,
And left him right-side blind.

So sailing's off, and driving too,
The 'Rosalind' is sold.
Now even memories are vague,
Those carefree days of old.

But here we are on Swing-bed Yacht
In Front Verandah Bay.
Great-grandson Judah's having fun,
New joys are his each day.

His merry laugh and sparkling eyes
Light up Great-granddad's smile,
There's expectation, life, and hope
In thirteenth great-grandchild.

Ralph leaves a heritage that's rich
And yachting's just a part.
He loved the Word – the Christ, the Book,
His compass, haven, heart.

But just for now old Captain Ralph
Nods off, with chin on chest,
Leave him to sleep in Swing-bed yacht
In trusting, child-like rest.

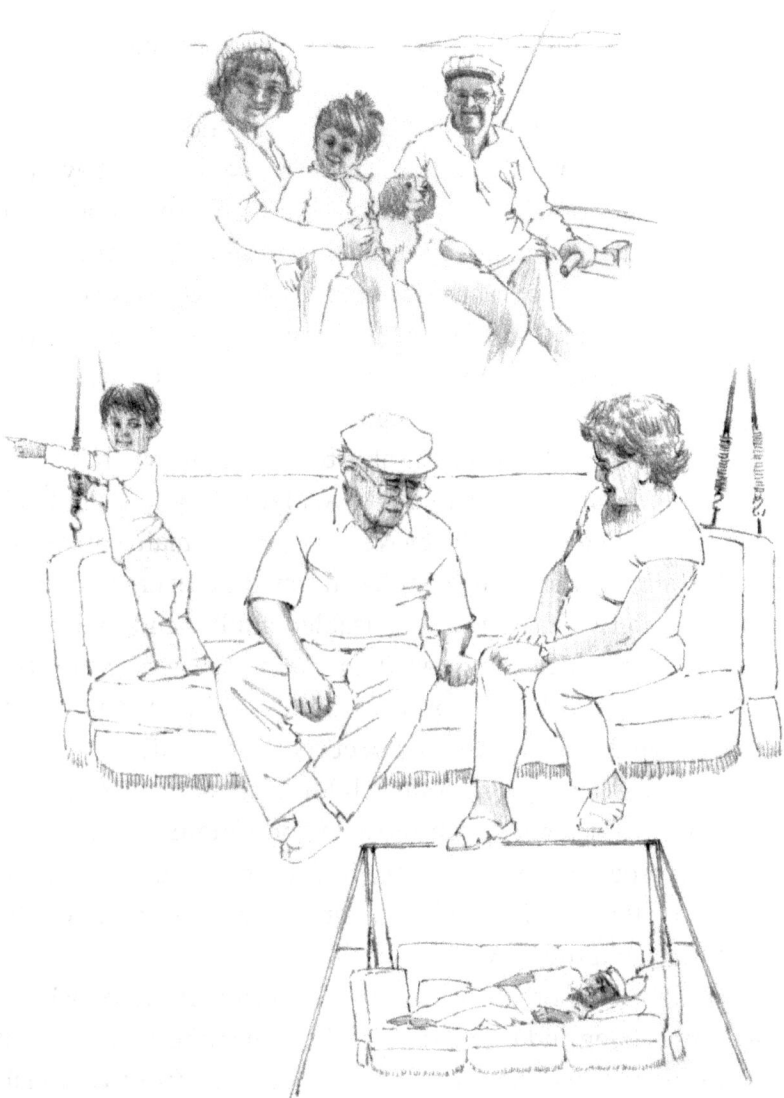

YACHTING HAD TRULY BEEN a much-loved part of Dad's life and he knew a great deal about sailing in the Waitemata Harbour, Hauraki Gulf and up the eastern coast north of Auckland. On one occasion, a friend brought a map of the harbour and was surprised at how animated Ralph became and how much he knew about the winds and currents in the various bays (an example of another 'primary theme' for Dad). In his later life he spent many hours sitting or lying on the swing-bed, gently rocking in the sun, perhaps thinking of his sailing days or even remembering back to the swing-bed which had been on the verandah of his childhood home in Ngataringa Rd, where his mother slept on hot summer nights!

So it was ideal that Dad was able to stay in his own home, living with his grandson David, his wife Marcelle, and their small children Judah and Zion. They were wonderful main caregivers for his last two and a half years. With David's university holiday work experience in homes for disabled adults, and Marcelle's years of nursing, nothing fazed them, (which was partly the inspiration behind 'Pooh Corner' – their good-hearted approach to the inevitable accidents that occurred with Dad).

Living in a family with young children created a lively, noisy atmosphere for Dad, which most of the time he didn't mind and often seemed to appreciate. It also offered me the opportunity to reflect on the similarities and differences between the very young and the very old.

'Swing-bed Yacht' arose out of a delightful afternoon when I was baby-sitting and Dad-sitting at the same time, and we spent some time together on the swing-bed on Dad's front verandah. We pretended it was a yacht, which stimulated Dad's memories of his yachting days, and gave Judah many opportunities to climb on and off and generally have fun. What a precious memory for me, which I tried to capture in the poem. Although Judah, about eighteen months old at the time, won't remember that golden experience, I am sure it blended into his life's tapestry to make him a fuller, richer person. There were two-way experiences going on in Dad's home; good satisfying interactions, the stuff that makes strong families and grows mutual care and understanding.

Life Day by Day

Pooh Corner

How are you today Dad?
Just How, he replies mournfully
– like Eeyore
But that's not why it's called Pooh Corner.

A little boy reads Winnie-the-Pooh
And there are rabbits and a soft toy
– just like Piglet
But that's not why it's called Pooh Corner.

Outside are wild bits of garden
With some thick juicy thistles and trees
– like 100 Acre Wood
But that's not why it's called Pooh Corner.

But here's a lovely little baby girl
And here's a busy lively toddler
And a great-grandfather who doesn't always make it in time
And – say no more –
    That's why it's called Pooh Corner!!

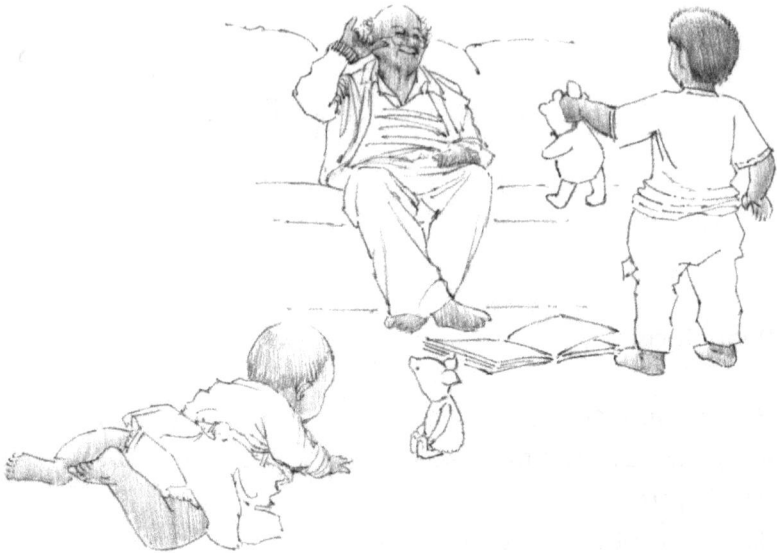

R<small>ALPH WAS AWARE</small> of the internal prompt to go to the toilet until a relatively short time before his death, and if all went well, would often get there in time. But for most people, incontinence eventually becomes a part of dementia, as it does for many older people without dementia too. There are many contributing factors, including less obvious ones like slow gait or losing one's way to the toilet. Accidents may be prevented by simple measures such as having the toilet relatively nearby, with a clear distinguishing sign on its door, and the toilet seat in a contrasting colour to the flooring and walls so it is easily seen. Night lights may guide the way to the toilet. Caregivers can prompt the person at regular intervals.

We are greatly assisted in New Zealand by nurses specialised in continence care who can give advice. Subsidised continence

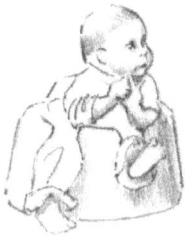

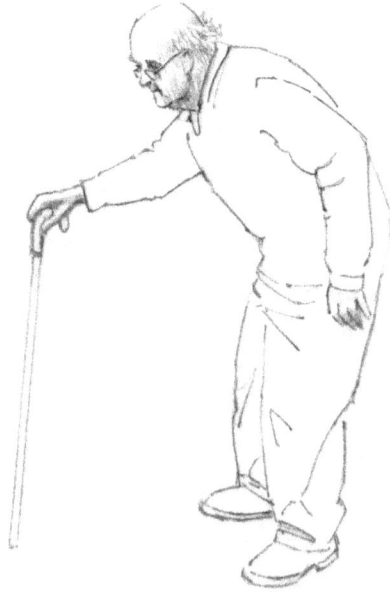

aids like pull-up adult diapers also make the problem much easier to deal with.

Sometimes a change in continence may indicate a temporary problem which can be treated, resulting in a return to the previous level of continence. Examples are urinary tract infection, prostate enlargement, dietary changes and infective or other forms of diarrhoea. Any little measure to keep the person continent is well worthwhile for the person's own dignity as well as for the convenience of the caregivers.

Simple Solutions

Walking slowly,
    Slowly... slowly,
        Long pause,
            Another step...
                Slowly... slower...

There's a step to navigate.
'Lift your foot, Daddy.'
'I can't.'
'Just lift it a little... the right one first.'
(I tug on his trouser leg to indicate which one.)
'I can't,' he says, irritated, and stands immobile.

(What's happening now?
Right leg weakness?
Stroke?
Parkinson's?)

Oh! His left foot is standing on the cuff of his right trouser leg!

It's always worth looking for the simple solution!

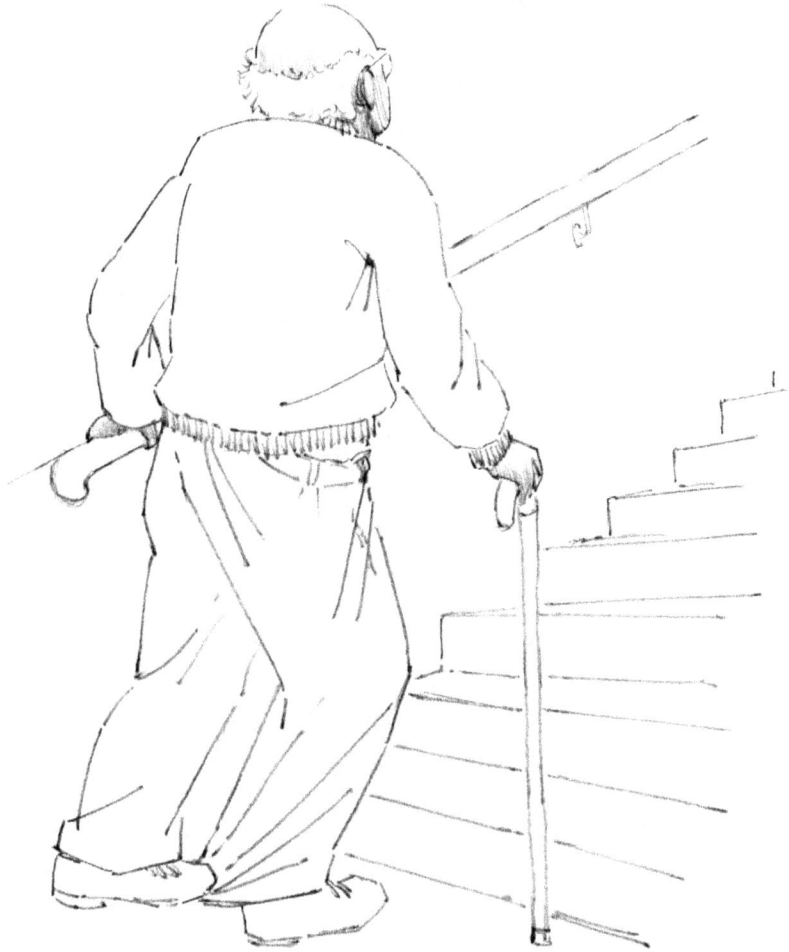

SEEMINGLY SMALL INTERVENTIONS can make relatively big differences for people with dementia; differences which may be positive or negative in their effect. Clearly in this example, Dad just needed his trousers shortened – an intervention that was important for his safety too. When the dining room table was shifted, it was noticed that if Dad got up to go to the toilet he would head off in the opposite direction. So his place was changed to the opposite side of the table and that corrected the problem. We also noticed that Dad would often finish eating with only half of his plate empty, the left half. Turning the plate around so that the rest of the food was on the left side worked better than cajoling him to eat more. This was of course because of his right-sided blindness, but his dementia prevented him from compensating for it.

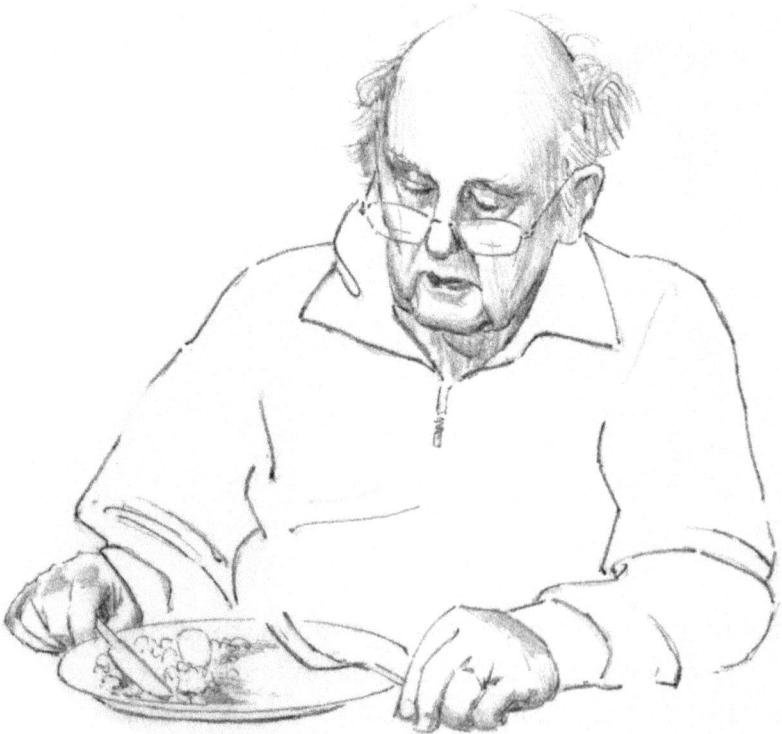

Thank You for Understanding

David gives Granddad his breakfast.
 Dad says, 'Thank you' and eats it
 but later he asks, 'Where's breakfast?'
  Thank you for understanding.

The 'Bath Lady' helps Ralph with his shower.
 Dad says, 'Thank you' though he
 grumbles his way to the bathroom!
  Thank you for understanding.

Marcelle puts Granddad's clothes away.
 Dad says, 'Thank you' but later
 he'll have no idea where they are.
  Thank you for understanding.

A friend takes Ralph to the movies.
 Dad says, 'Thank you' but sleeps right through
 and won't recall a thing of it.
  Thank you for understanding.

I play old hymns on the piano.
 Dad sings a little and says, 'Thank you'
 but he won't remember our evening.

(And I'm so out of practice.
Thank you, Dad, for understanding!)

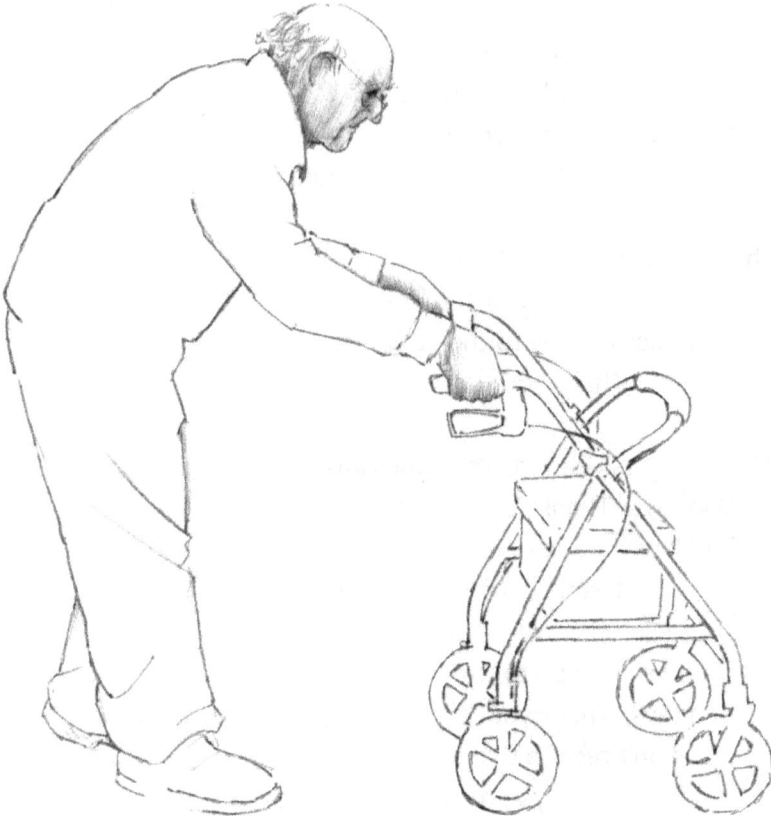

As PEOPLE WITH DEMENTIA have to come to grips with their new selves (and how much insight they actually have can be hard to know), so too must the caregivers. Caring for a family member with dementia is hard, repetitive, fraught with highs and lows, and at times apparently thankless. It is particularly difficult when it falls mainly to just one individual. That one caregiver can't help wondering, 'Does this person have any idea how much I do, how much my sleep is disturbed, how sometimes I just want to run away?' Yet many caregivers can testify to the expressions of affection and appreciation which come their way from time to time. My father said thank you often, and although he was not very expressive in the way he said it, I have a sense that he genuinely appreciated the care he was receiving. It would show in the little hand squeeze, the pat on the back, or the occasional wink or smile. Teaching children to say thank you, and making it a habit, can have positive repercussions down through the years, way beyond what we anticipate at the start. Saying thank you can keep a person going!

Habits

Long held habits last longest –
    like locking the front door at night,
    turning off the lights on leaving the room,
    washing hands after using the toilet,
    saying thank you for kindnesses, and
    Bible memory verses!

Today,
    dementia far advanced,
        Dad depressed, dragging on,
            dawdling through his meals
                sighing, groaning, eyes closed, miserable.
Then, he said it, John 14 verse 6[18]
'I am the way, and the truth, and the life.
No-one comes to the Father except through me.'

Startling, arresting, those words Jesus said,
those words Dad said –
Today.

It's in there,
in his brain,
stowed away as a lad,
repeated many times
and today, amazingly, dug out
to shed hope upon his way –
Today.

_____

18. John 14:6, *The Bible.*

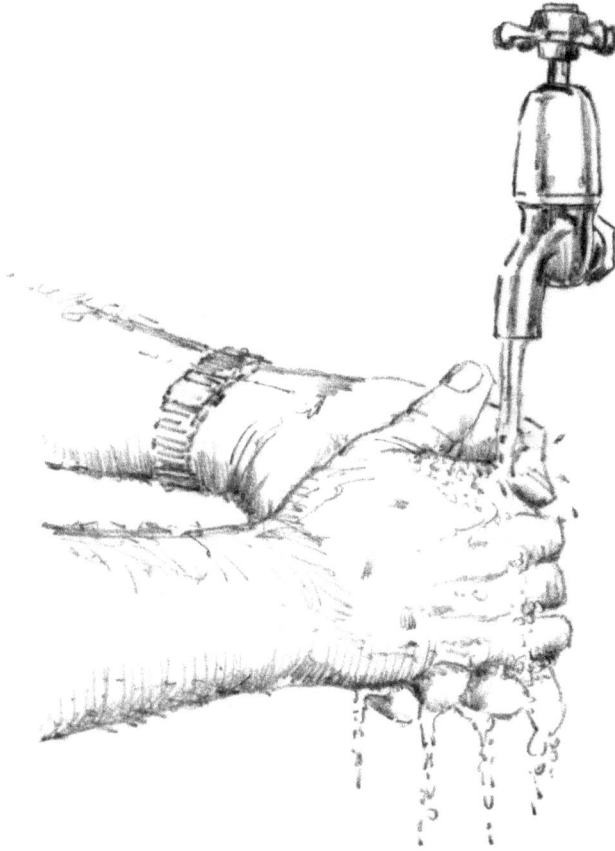

HABITS, LIKE THE FACETS of personality and the knowledge and skills learned and practised over many years, persist well into dementia, no doubt lasting longer the earlier they were formed – like saying thank you. Ralph's sister Ainslie told the story she had heard from her mother of when Ralph, as a preschooler, visited the lady next door. He returned to tell his mother about the piece of cake he had been given, adding '...and I said please and ta!'

Such habits may soften the impact of what is happening to a loved family member. Simple practical habits like washing hands are very helpful for obvious reasons, and saying thank you oils relationships and makes life more pleasant. Sometimes habits may be repeated almost obsessively. Early in Dad's dementia he would repeatedly check that the front door was locked, opening and relocking it, even during the night. The live-in caregiver at the time became nervous that in his confusion he would leave the door open or lock himself outside. As with many aspects of dementia, a simple intervention can often help. In this case a sign – DOOR LOCKED – was hung on the door handle at night and the key hidden. Dad seemed to get the message.

There are people with dementia in whom unpleasant habits are prominent and indeed appear to become exaggerated as the years go by. Everyone finds it difficult to care for a domineering, complaining older relative. We were blessed to have a father who had, in most areas of his life, become gentler and easier to be with.

Pill Power

It's amazing what a tiny pill can do!
For a while there, Dad was very agitated,
 Wakeful at night,
 Calling out,
'Ahoy there!'   'Anybody there?'
We were up several times a night.
New caregivers were due to arrive,
They had a little baby.
They didn't want two 'babies' disturbing their nights!

So he was given risperidone at night,
Just a tiny dose,
And it made a big difference,
He began to sleep better.

But the repetition continued,
Phrases, words, questions or snatches of a song.
'Amen' with an upward lilt was one of them,
Repeated inappropriately – but never in church, funnily enough –
And easily mimicked by younger family members.
Earlier it had been 'Puhoi',
Perhaps dragged up from old memories of sailing up that river.[19]
The little bursts of a hymn tune were pleasanter,
But even they began to grate on us.

---

19. Puhoi is a settlement located approximately 50km north of
Auckland, New Zealand, on the banks of the Puhoi River.

I'm Ralph, I'm Dad

And he still seemed so unhappy.
'Might as well cut my head off,' he'd say;
'I'm just a silly old cow.'
He'd sit slumped in a chair,
Lightly scratching his bald pate,
Irritated by the baby noises of his great-grandson.
Was he depressed?
He was still confused about where Mum had gone.
He thought we hadn't told him she was dying.

So we visited the geriatrician
And the decision was made.
He'll take another little pill, an antidepressant.
Within a very few days the effect was apparent –
no more repetition
no more negative comments about himself
much less sitting scratching his head
increased interest in the great-grandson.

It was amazing!
It was wonderful!
It was scary!

Such tiny pills! Such a dramatic result!
Such an effect on someone's brain, on his mind.
How would it affect a 'normal' brain?
What about all the difficult, irritating people in society?
        Mind control?
        Population control?

Pill power!

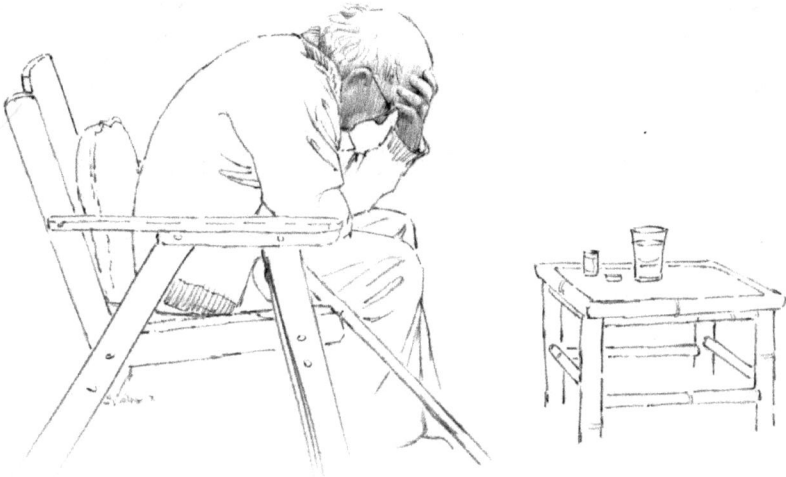

THE USE OF MEDICATION in dementia always needs to be approached with caution, but it can have an amazing, and apparently very positive effect. I say 'apparently' because I sometimes wondered if the medication, especially the risperidone prescribed for agitation, closed Dad down in a way, and prevented us having access into little windows of his mind which we might not otherwise have known about.

The incident referred to in 'Ralph's In' occurred one night when he was in a restless stage, not long before he started risperidone. It was an episode in which he was agitated and upset, and which disturbed my sleep but at the same time gave me an insight into a period of his life when he took part in school sports. It was a precious little gem of his past, not previously known to me, and I wonder if more would have been revealed if he hadn't started taking risperidone.

73

So, prescribing medications for the symptoms of dementia is a balancing act between assisting with the care of the person, providing comfort and ease, without creating a chemical straitjacket. For more on the use of medicines in dementia, including medicines for depression which can often occur but be difficult to distinguish from the dementia, see Appendix 7.

Winding Down

Half Missing

Married *sixty years*!
    And in our modern times, we wonder.

Married *sixty years*!
    And our age of cheap replacements asks, how?
        And, what good does it do?
           And, why would you want to?

Amazed, we look at an old man,
    An old man with dementia.

One wife for sixty years
Until they knew each other back to front,
Shared homes and gardens
    Yachts and camping
    Books and chess
    Kids and grandkids
    Struggles and joys.

I'm Ralph, I'm Dad

A solid life experience of love and acceptance
A bedrock of faithfulness and trust
A mystery of one flesh
That only death would finally invade
    And tear apart
        And leave a man – half missing
Yet not lost, for in his final days
        Ralph still recalled his Hazel and was comforted.

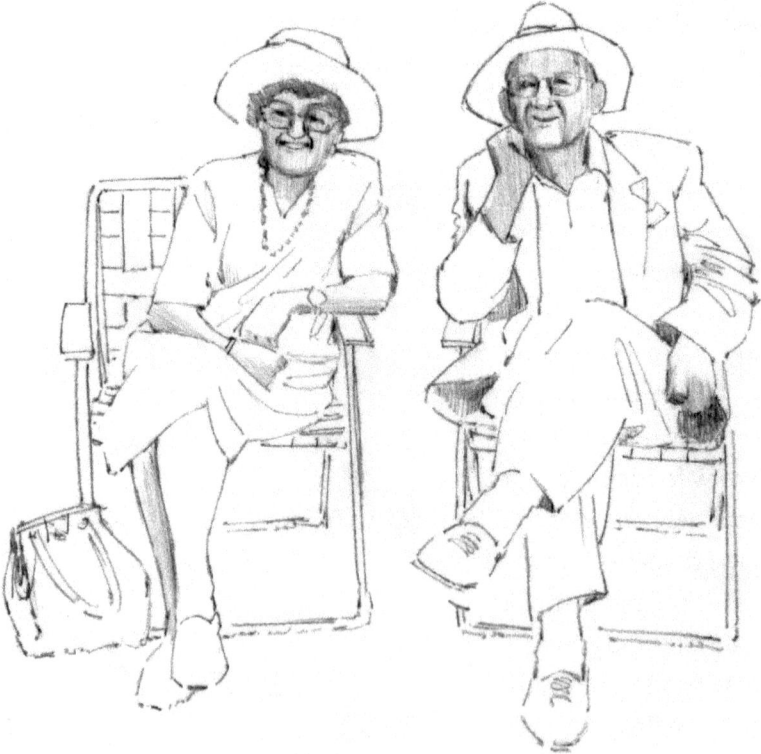

I HAVE OFTEN WONDERED what was going on in a marriage like that of my parents. They were totally committed to marriage being lifelong, 'for better or for worse', fully respecting the Biblical statement that 'a man will leave his father and mother and be united to his wife, and they will become one flesh'.[20]

Thinking about their long marriage, and in contrast, the huge trauma often suffered by married or de facto couples who separate – a trauma which may affect physical health as well as mental and spiritual wellbeing – I am convinced that the 'one flesh' is more than a poetic phrase or a politely veiled reference to sexual intimacy. Losing one's friend and partner of many years can be compared to losing a limb – it hurts, disables, is missed, and is sometimes mistakenly felt to still be there! I remember one elderly gentleman with dementia who would repeatedly wander off looking for his deceased wife, eventually requiring that he live in a secure dementia unit.

My father couldn't take it in that Mum wasn't going to come home from the hospital. Even though her body lay in a coffin at home the night before her funeral, and even though he attended her funeral and burial, he couldn't retain the memory that she had died. He would ask us when she was going to come home and why we hadn't told him how sick she was. He couldn't express his sorrow clearly, but his depression and his occasional poignant comments indicated that he was indeed noticing the loss of his long-time companion. Once, when reminded it was Mum's birthday, he asked where she was. On being told she had died two years before he said, 'Oh, so that's who I've been missing.'

---

20. Genesis 2:24, *The Bible*, also quoted by Jesus Christ (Matthew 19:5) and Paul the Apostle (Ephesians 5:31).

For a long time he would enjoy looking at their wedding photo, recognising that he was the groom and she was his bride. 'That's my little Hazel,' he would say with a smile. But as his dementia progressed, memories of Mum appeared to fade. (Is that an 'advantage' of dementia – that one doesn't have to keep on processing those difficult memories?) But in his last few weeks both my sister and I had the bittersweet experience of Dad mistaking us for Mum. It was as if his 'little Hazel' who had been his faithful companion for so many years was with him right to the end.

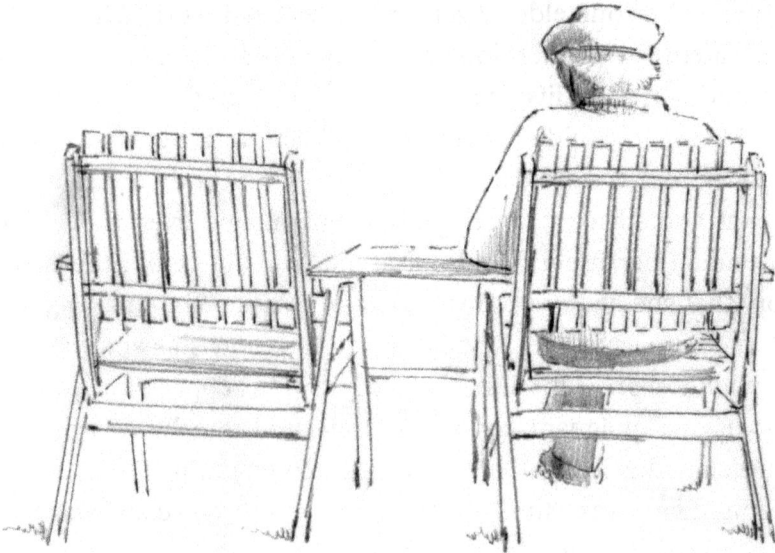

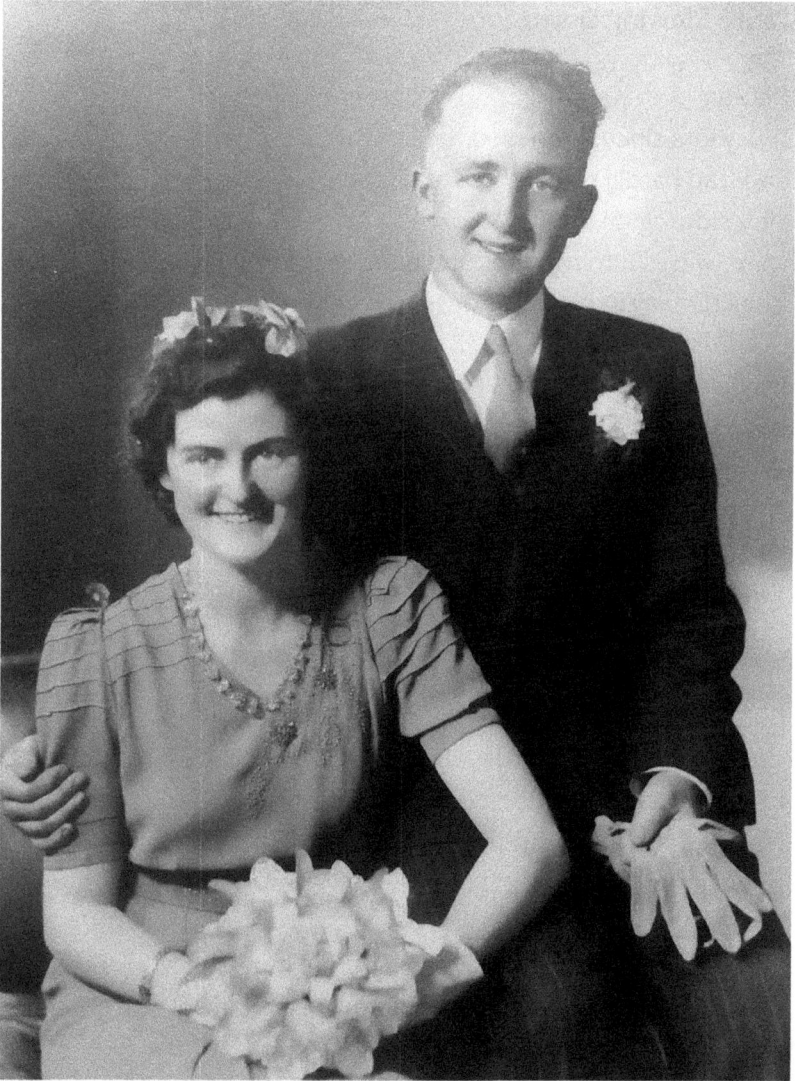

Hazel and Ralph on their wedding day.

Dad's Slowing Down

May 29th
Two years since Mum died,
and Dad hardly remembers his Hazel.
He's slowing down –
walks with shuffling steps and bent back,
loses his way in his own house.

It's Sunday morning, so I play some old hymns,
but all I get are a few little snatches.
'What a friend we have in Jesus...' – that's all.
A rumbling bass harmony now and then
            – or was it a snore?
'What about "All Hail the Power of Jesus' Name," Dad?'
'Number One', he replies – and yes, he's right!

But he's slowing down.

I ask him about his memories of the past,
his thoughts of the future,
but I get no response.

I read a verse of hope: 'May the God of Hope
fill you with all joy and peace as you trust in him,
so you may overflow with hope
by the power of the Holy Spirit.'[21]
but he says nothing.

---

21. Romans 15:13, *The Bible*.

Would you like to pray, Dad?
He starts his usual formula –
'Loving Heavenly Father
we thank you for your many blessings
that you provide us with from day to day
and we pray that we may...'
    His train of thought is lost, sleep overwhelms.
I whisper, 'God of Hope, we trust you',
...resume my hymn playing ...and blow my nose.

Yes, Dad's really slowing down now.

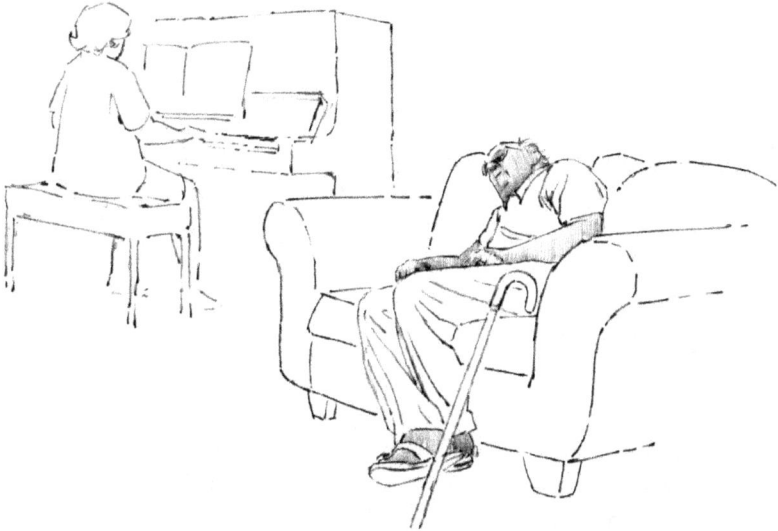

Ralph's In!

Ralph's in! He's run the race!
He's got to write his name on Taka's board.[22]
    Come on Dad – it's the early hours,
    You haven't run for years.

The old man is confused.
In the night, old memories take on weird reality.
The bedroom wall becomes the board,
But where's the pen?
He's agitated, even angry.
No use saying it was all a dream.
I give him a pencil
    And he writes on the wall –
        Taka
            Ralph's in
                1st in

He calms down, settles back in bed.
The curtain falls over the writing.

---

22. 'Taka' was how he wrote Takapuna; he had attended Takapuna
Grammar School. This incident happened early in 2007, not long
before he was started on risperidone. His sister Ainslie explained the
story and why it may have stuck in his mind. After he had written his
name on the board as the first runner to arrive, the boy who came
second put his name ahead of Ralph's so Ralph did not get honoured
as first place-getter. Not one to make a fuss, he just absorbed the
injustice, only, it appears, for it to rise up and come out at this time
when his brain was rearranging itself.

Ralph's run his race,
  His name's on the board,
    He's in the winning team!

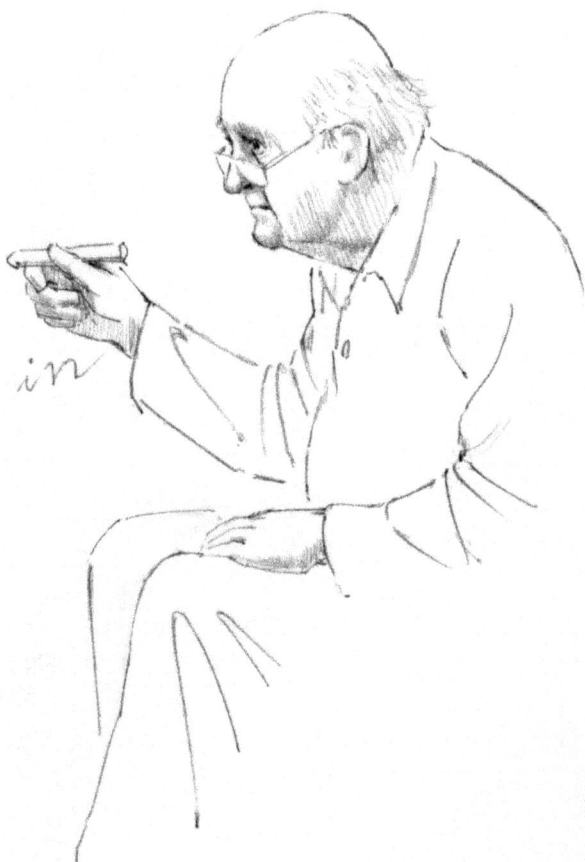

In Church

Dear Dad, you stand in church,
    You teach the Word divine
    You sing with strong bass voice
    You bless the bread and wine.

Dear Dad, you sit in church,
    You lean on stick, head bowed
    As unknown songs swirl round,
    Alone within the crowd.

Dear Dad, you wait at home,
    Quote verses memorised,
    You sing the old loved hymns
    You pray, Spirit inspired.

Dear Dad, you lie in church
    Our memories we confide,
    We voice our heartfelt thanks,
    Sleep now by Hazel's side.

'I have fought the good fight, I have finished the race, I have kept the faith. Now there is in store for me the crown of righteousness, which the Lord, the righteous Judge will award me on that day – and not only me but also to all who have longed for his appearing.'[23]

---

23. 2 Timothy 4:7-8, *The Bible*.

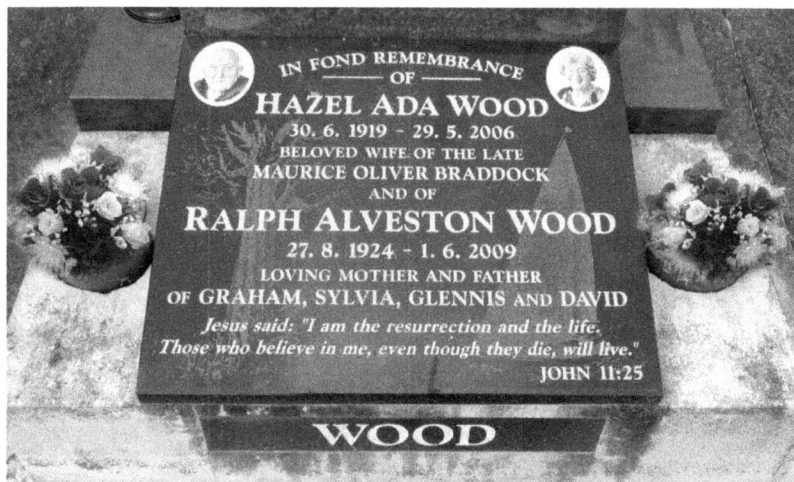

As Dad's dementia progressed, we often marvelled at the persistence of his Christian faith, that supremely important facet of his life. When he had forgotten almost everything else, including short and long-term memories and the identity of family members, fragments of old hymns, Bible verses and prayers still came to the fore. Indeed towards the end (April 2009), they surfaced even more clearly than the confused nonsense statements we had noted previously. We took to reading well-known Bible passages to him, pausing at key words, and he usually filled them in correctly. When I said I would read Psalm 23 to him, he immediately responded, 'The Lord is my Shepherd.' (See Appendix 8 for a comment on spirituality in dementia.)

As most of his mental capacity was stripped away, it was a comfort for us, and hopefully for him, to know that he had been left with the solid bedrock of his faith in God and the precious promises of the Bible. It seemed to us that for Dad, dementia had 'Dealt Gently', and he was indeed 'held in the memories of God'.[24]

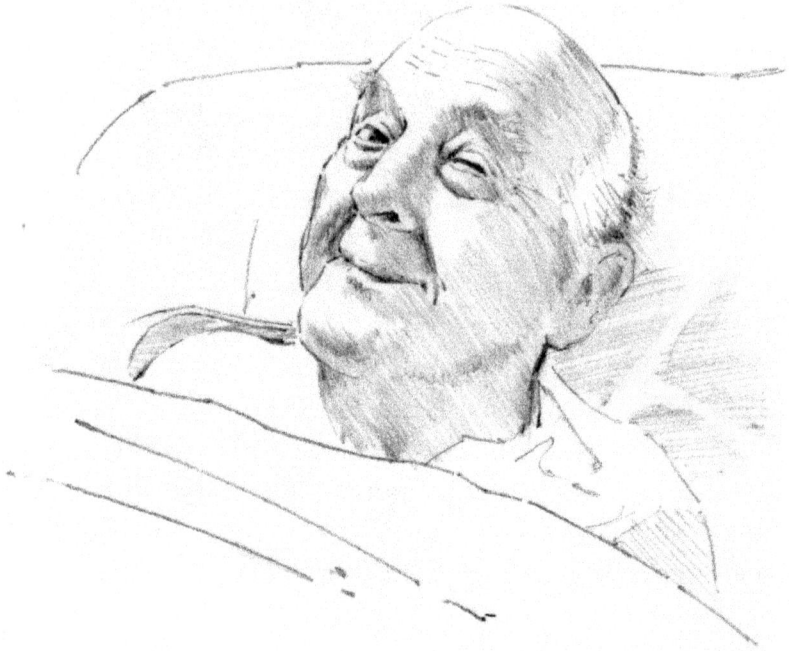

---

24. Swinton, *Dementia: Living in the Memories of God*, p.211. 'God is mindful of human beings. To be human is to be held in the memory of God. God watches over human beings, knows them intimately, and remembers them.'

Appendices

Appendix 1: Definition of dementia

'DEMENTIA IS A SYNDROME – usually of a chronic or progressive nature – in which there is deterioration in cognitive function (i.e. the ability to process thought) beyond what might be expected from normal ageing. It affects memory, thinking, orientation, comprehension, calculation, learning capacity, language, and judgement. Consciousness is not affected. The impairment in cognitive function is commonly accompanied, and occasionally preceded, by deterioration in emotional control, social behaviour, or motivation. Dementia results from a variety of diseases and injuries that primarily or secondarily affect the brain, such as Alzheimer's disease or stroke.'[25]

Dementia is caused by damage to or loss of nerve cells and their connections in the brain. Depending on the area of the brain that's affected by the damage, dementia can affect people differently and cause different symptoms. Alzheimer's disease is the most common cause of dementia. Vascular dementia is the second most common type of dementia and is caused by

---

25. World Health Organisation, September 2019, www.who.int/news-room/fact-sheets/detail/dementia.

damage to the vessels that supply blood to the brain. Blood vessel problems can cause strokes or damage the brain in other ways.[26]

Appendix 2: Dementia: early signs and other conditions

THE EARLY STAGE OF DEMENTIA can be difficult to detect, with subtle changes in behaviour, personality, orientation (e.g. getting mixed up about date and place), and short term memory loss. All of these changes fluctuate and the caring family member or observer, or the person experiencing symptoms, will have trouble initially putting their finger on what, if anything, is going on. Forgetfulness may put a person or their property at risk, for example, by leaving a frying pan on the stove so it catches fire or forgetting to lock the house at night. Events like this may be the trigger to seek a diagnosis. At this early stage, the person may lack insight into what they are doing, or they may be aware and embarrassed and try to cover up for 'mistakes'. Some may become very defensive and even suspicious when concerned people try to intervene. This can be a very worrying and difficult time for family and friends.

Later, especially in Alzheimer's type dementia, people can be quite restless and agitated. They may wander off and get lost. Caregivers have the difficult task of restricting freedom for the person's own safety, while at the same time showing respect and kindness and allowing interest and variety in the person's life.

Mobility problems and bladder incontinence commonly

---

26. Mayo Clinic, *Dementia*, 19 April 2019, www.mayoclinic.org/diseases-conditions/dementia/symptoms-causes/syc-20352013.

appear in dementia as it progresses, but they can also be early signs of a rare kind of dementia caused by normal pressure hydrocephalus. It is worth diagnosing early because there is a surgical intervention which often reverses the process or slows progression, if it is carried out early.

Being passive and inactive is a feature of dementia which tends to occur more in vascular type dementia, but it can also be an indication of depression or of some other medical condition such as an underactive thyroid gland (hypothyroidism) or a low level of vitamin B12, either alone or in combination with dementia. Both of these can be easily confirmed by a blood test and treated with replacement of the thyroxine hormone or vitamin B12. If started early enough, these treatments can reverse many of the observed features of these conditions. Depression also can be treated, sometimes with medication, but more importantly by appropriate interaction with supportive, interested people.

Appendix 3: What is the cause of dementia and can it be treated or prevented?[27]

THE ANSWER TO THESE QUESTIONS is the subject of much research, and no doubt understanding will change as new find-

---

27. Much of this material on risk factors is taken from the Fischer Centre for Alzheimer's Research Foundation: www.alzinfo.org, and Alzheimer's New Zealand: www.alzheimers.org.nz. The Alzheimer's NZ website is easier to navigate for non-medical people. A simple Google search will lead to numerous other websites which provide much information about all aspects and types of dementia.

ings come out, but some points are commonly accepted and helpful. The general answer is that many factors contribute to the complex processes which result in dementia. Increasing age is the strongest risk factor although, less commonly, the disease can occur at a younger age – under sixty-five.

Alzheimer's dementia[28] appears to be in part a genetic condition, meaning that there is a higher risk of developing it if there is a family history of Alzheimer's dementia, although even this is far from confirmed. However, some other diseases may contribute to the development of dementia. Stroke[29] is one of the most common of these, and behind that, all the problems that make stroke more likely to happen, such as high blood pressure, diabetes, high fats in the blood and smoking. Excessive alcohol intake over many years may be involved in the development of dementia. Other possibly reversible causes are certain drugs, an underactive thyroid gland, insufficient vitamin B12, depression, low blood pressure, poor diabetes control, some infections and even dehydration. Strictly speaking, some of these treatable conditions may actually cause delirium, which is a reversible form of confusion often mimicking dementia but also sometimes drawing attention to an underlying early dementia. Head injury after a fall with bleeding under the skull can cause a

---

28. Alzheimer's Dementia is the most common form, accounting for 50 to 70 percent of cases.

29. Vascular dementia accounts for 20 to 30 percent of cases and is caused by poor blood supply to the brain as a result of a stroke or several mini-strokes, or by the slow accumulation of blood vessel disease in the brain. Vascular dementia symptoms can begin suddenly after a stroke or gradually as disease in the blood vessels worsens. Some people will have both vascular dementia and Alzheimer's disease (Source: Alzheimer's New Zealand).

dementia-like situation which is reversible by removal of the blood which is pressing on the brain. Brain tumour and normal pressure hydrocephalus are other rare causes of dementia which may be treatable. Parkinson's and some other neurological (nerve) diseases may be associated with specific forms of dementia (Lewy body dementia and normal pressure hydrocephalus) which have more prominent mobility problems such as frequent falls or balance issues. Low levels of education and experiences early in life (including brain injury which has apparently resolved) may contribute to the complex processes which result in dementia.

Dietary habits may also play a part. Studies are bringing in evidence that a diet rich in foods containing vitamin E (such as vegetable oils, nuts, green leafy vegetables, and whole grains) may help protect against Alzheimer's in some people, a protective effect not seen when study participants simply took vitamin E supplements. A low-fat, antioxidant-rich diet containing at least five servings a day of fruits and vegetables is associated with decreased risk of Alzheimer's disease. Other studies have shown possible links between Alzheimer's dementia and deficiencies of vitamin B12 and folic acid. A diet rich in omega-3 fatty acids found in fish, seeds and nuts, has been linked to heart and brain health. Eating wisely throughout one's life and limiting alcohol consumption to a very small amount of red wine appears to be just as important to long-term brain health as it is to heart health.

Keeping mentally and physically active right through life, with lots of social activities, also appears to be protective. 'Not all activities are equal in this regard. Those that involve genuine concentration – studying a musical instrument, playing board games, reading and dancing – are associated with a lower risk for dementia. Dancing, which requires learning new moves, is both physically and mentally challenging and requires much concentration... Physical activity is helpful not only because it creates new neurones [nerve cells] but because the mind is based in the brain, and the brain needs oxygen. Walking, cycling, or cardiovascular exercise strengthens the heart and the blood vessels that supply the brain and helps people who engage in these activities feel mentally sharper...'[30]

Of course, increasing age is the strongest risk factor for dementia, and women seem to succumb with greater frequency than men, but that may be because they tend to live longer.

Supporting much of the above are observations of healthy, long-lived people who have been found to reside in what have been called 'Blue Zones' – five identified yet widespread geographic areas. They are Okinawa (Japan), Sardinia (Italy), Nicoya Peninsula (Costa Rica), Icaria (Greece) and among the Seventh-day Adventists in Loma Linda, California. Not only do people live longer in these areas, they also lead healthier, more active lives into their nineties and past the age of one hundred. They have lower incidence of many chronic diseases of older age, including dementia. Much has been written about why they have such long healthy lives, and a quick Google search for Blue Zones shows a huge range of information. One of the earliest and most well-respected books is *The Blue Zones: Lessons for Living Longer from the People Who've Lived the Longest* by Dan Buettner.[31]

---

30. Norman Doidge, MD, *The Brain that Changes Itself*, Carlton North, Vic.: Scribe Publications, 2008, pp.254 & 255.

31. Dan Buettner, *The Blue Zones: Lessons for Living Longer from the People Who've Lived the Longest*, Washington, D.C.: National Geographic, 2008. p.vii.

He provides a list of nine lessons, covering the lifestyle of blue zones people:

1. Moderate, regular physical activity
2. Life purpose
3. Stress reduction
4. Moderate calories intake
5. Plant-based diet
6. Moderate alcohol intake, especially wine
7. Engagement in spirituality or religion
8. Engagement in family life
9. Engagement in social life.[32]

Appendix 4: Does losing your memory really make you a non-person?

COLLEEN CARROLL CAMPBELL states the fear of dementia well: 'The oblivion and dependence that dementia brings on are frightening prospects in a culture that exalts reason and autonomy, and often uses both to define our status as persons.'[33]

But she also comes to some encouraging conclusions, including this: 'Alzheimer's disease exposes the flaws inherent in locating the self exclusively in the mind and assuming that only those with awareness and memory are persons. As ethicist Gilbert Meilaender wrote recently, in a paper presented to his

---

32. Taken from en.wikipedia.org/wiki/Blue_Zone but there are many more relevant websites.

33. Colleen Carroll Campbell, 'The Human Face of Alzheimer's', *The New Atlantis*, Number 6, Summer 2004, p.7.

colleagues on the President's Council on Bioethics, 'one might take the living body, not the immaterial will or the power of choice, as the locus of personal presence.' We are not minds alone or bodies alone, but 'embodied souls' and 'ensouled bodies.' To understand this truth is to understand the dignity of those whose minds are fading, but whose presence as persons can never be in doubt. Those with Alzheimer's disease remind us most vividly that our humanity comprises both our bodies and our minds, and perhaps something else that transcends them both.'[34]

Swinton's chapter on 'Personhood and Humanness' is also helpful in understanding that personhood isn't just to do with having certain capacities but is inherent in being a human being. 'Personhood thus relates to the way that human beings are in the world and relate in and to one another and the world. It is not a set of capacities, and it is not simply a standing that is bestowed on someone by others. It is an irrevocable status that comes from being a human being.'[35]

Appendix 5: Making a present of the past

PENNY GARNER, a UK housewife who by observation and clever trial and error developed a now well-recognised system of patient-centred care called SPECIAL (Specialised Early Care for Alzheimer's), has taken the idea of photographs to quite a different level.[36] She thinks of memories as photos stored in a

---

34. Campbell, 'The Human Face of Alzheimer's', p.10.

35. Swinton, *Dementia: Living in the Memories of God*, p.157.

36. Penny Garner's story and a clear description of SPECIAL and

photo album with the actual facts of the 'photo' as well as the feelings associated with that memory. In someone with dementia, recent 'photos' are not stored well, but carers can find out what were the old 'photos' that had happy or satisfying feelings associated with them and then use those to create 'a present of the past' and with it a much more contented person than has often been the case for sufferers of dementia.

Appendix 6: Using photos to stave off memory loss

WENDY MITCHELL received her diagnosis of dementia early in its course when she was in her fifties and still working, and because of this, she was able to do many things to adapt to her new self. Labelling photos while she still remembered what and who they were, and then pegging them up on strings in her spare room to create a 'memory room', was her way of preserving the memories represented by the photos. She also realised, like Penny Garner (Appendix 5), that the feelings associated with a photo can be retained even if the names and details of the photo have been forgotten.

Appendix 7: Medicines in dementia

THERE IS NO 'MAGIC BULLET' yet which can cure or reverse dementia, but there are a few medicines which may improve symptoms of the disease for a while. One group of medications

---

how to use it in the care of people with dementia is told in James, *Contented Dementia*. See p.41ff for the photograph album.

called cholinesterase inhibitors has shown limited usefulness in slowing the progression of early dementia. They have been studied mainly in Alzheimer's type dementia but have shown some effectiveness in other forms of dementia too. Another drug called memantine works a little differently and also alleviates the expression of dementia for a while, possibly around six months in some people. Side effects may limit the use of all these drugs.[37] Even a short gain may allow people with dementia and their families to put in place decisions about enduring power of attorney, the signing off of a will and advanced care planning. Ideally, however, these important tasks are best done well in advance of the development of dementia.

---

37. New Zealand Formulary release 91, 1 Jan 2020, 4.11:v91. Medicines may be used as an adjunct to non-pharmacological treatment. When medicines are used they should be initiated in consultation with a specialist team experienced in the management of dementia. Treatment should be reassessed on a regular basis and continued only when considered to be having a worthwhile effect on symptoms. Donepezil hydrochloride, galantamine and rivastigmine (acetylcholinesterase inhibitors) are recommended for the treatment of cognitive symptoms of mild-to-moderate dementia due to Alzheimer's disease. Memantine hydrochloride is a suitable alternative for patients with moderate-to-severe Alzheimer's disease when acetylcholinesterase inhibitors are contraindicated or are not tolerated... Acetylcholinesterase inhibitors can cause unwanted dose-related cholinergic effects (most commonly gastro-intestinal effects such as nausea, vomiting, diarrhoea, dyspepsia; urinary incontinence; dizziness). They should be started at a low dose and increased according to tolerability. Choice of agent is generally determined by cost, mode of delivery and risk of adverse effects; there is no evidence that one acetylcholinesterase inhibitor is more effective than the others... Acetylcholinesterase inhibitors have been associated with heart block and sinus bradycardia.

Agitation and sleeping difficulties are common in dementia and very small doses of the atypical antipsychotics can often be helpful.

Depression occurs in 20 to 40 percent of cases of dementia and is more common early on and in vascular dementia, or if there have been previous problems with depression. It can be difficult to diagnose because many of the symptoms of depression such as apathy, loss of interest, poor appetite, and sleep disturbance may also be features of dementia. Providing a stimulating, interesting and caring environment, sometimes with counselling, may be helpful in treating depression but there is also a place for antidepressant medication and it certainly seemed to have a very positive effect on Ralph. He was able to take more interest in what was going on around him and be less tough on himself – which had a good effect on the caregivers too! A geriatrician was involved at this time, because adding drugs that work in the brain to the medication regime of a person with dementia can be fraught with difficulties and requires expert knowledge and experience on the part of the prescriber. Many people are on an array of tablets for pre-existing chronic diseases and the more medicines they take, the greater the risk of interactions and unpleasant or dangerous side-effects.

Appendix 8: Spirituality in dementia

MANY RESEARCHERS AND OBSERVERS of dementia, including those with Alzheimer's dementia themselves, have noted the importance of spiritual aspects in this progressive disease, not only to cope with it but to understand and rise above it. Colleen Carroll Campbell, a fellow at the Ethics and Public Policy

Center in Washington DC, in her article 'The Human Face of Alzheimer's' notes: 'The heightened spiritual sense that follows a dementia diagnosis often lingers long after other memories and impressions have faded. Even those in the advanced stages of Alzheimer's may remain remarkably lucid about core religious beliefs and retain an almost intuitive knowledge of the religious rituals that shaped their lives. Caregivers tell stories of severely demented loved ones who no longer know the names of their children or where they are, but still recite flawless rosaries, sing rousing renditions of 'Amazing Grace,' or respond with reverence during the candle lighting that ushers in the Jewish Sabbath.'

Professor John Swinton's book, *Dementia: Living in the Memories of God*, brings this out in fascinating detail, with many references to examples and research. He challenges caregivers, family, and others to think again about what is going on in dementia and how we should respond to it.

Bibliography

Buettner, Dan. *The Blue Zones: Lessons for Living Longer from the People Who've Lived the Longest.* Washington, D.C.: National Geographic, 2008.

Campbell, Colleen Carroll. 'The Human Face of Alzheimer's'. *The New Atlantis 6.* Summer 2004.

Doidge, Norman. *The Brain that Changes Itself.* Carlton North, Vic.: Scribe Publications, 2008.

James, Oliver. *Contented Dementia.* London: Vermilion, 2008.

Mayo Clinic. *Dementia.* 19 April 2019. www.mayoclinic.org/diseases-conditions/dementia/symptoms-causes/syc-20352013.

Mitchell, Wendy, and Wharton, Anna. *Somebody I Used to Know.* London: Bloomsbury, 2018.

Swinton, John. *Dementia: Living in the Memories of God.* Grand Rapids, MI: W.B. Eerdmans, 2012.

Welch, Edward T. *Blame it on the Brain?* Phillipsburg, N.J.: Presbyterian & Reformed Publishing, 1998.

World Health Organisation. *Dementia.* 19 September 2019. www.who.int/news-room/fact-sheets/detail/dementia.

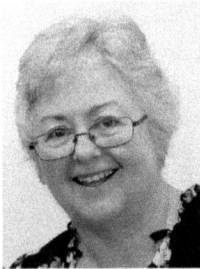

GLENNIS MAFI (MB ChB, FRNZCGP) was a doctor for 45 years, most of them in general practice in Tonga and Auckland. She retired in November 2019. She has both academic and personal experience of dementia, completing a Postgraduate Diploma in Geriatrics and helping to care for her father through his dementia. She is married to Manu and they have four married children and twelve grandchildren.

Contact Glennis by emailing glennis.books@gmail.com

www.ingramcontent.com/pod-product-compliance
Lightning Source LLC
Chambersburg PA
CBHW072107040426
42334CB00042B/2540